MC

Int

Medicine

GW01464812

Fourth Edition

2184 Single Choice MCQs with Answers

MCQs *in*

Internal
Medicine

Fourth Edition

2184 Single Choice MCQs with Answers

Arup Kumar Kundu MD, FICP, MNAS

Professor, Department of Medicine, and
In-charge, Division of Rheumatology
KPC Medical College, Kolkata
West Bengal, India

e-mail: arup_kundu@hotmail.com

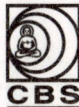

CBS

CBS Publishers & Distributors Pvt Ltd
New Delhi • Bengaluru • Chennai • Kochi • Pune
Hyderabad • Kolkata • Manipal • Mumbai • Nagpur • Patna

MCQs *in*
Internal
Medicine
Fourth Edition

ISBN: 978-81-239-2256-0

Copyright © Author and Publisher

Fourth Edition: 2013
First Edition: 2003
Second Edition: 2006
Third Edition: 2009

Published by Satish Kumar Jain for
CBS Publishers & Distributors Pvt Ltd
4819/XI Prahlad Street, 24 Ansari Road, Daryaganj, New Delhi 110 002, India.
Ph: 23289259, 23266861, 23266867   Fax: 011-23243014   Website: www.cbspd.com
e-mail: delhi@cbspd.com; cbspubs@airtelmail.in
Corporate Office: 204 FIE, Industrial Area, Patparganj, Delhi 110 092
Ph: 4934 4934   Fax: 4934 4935   e-mail: publishing@cbspd.com; publicity@cbspd.com

Branches

- **Bengaluru:** Seema House 2975, 17th Cross, K.R. Road,
  Banasankari 2nd Stage, Bengaluru 560 070, Karnataka
  Ph: +91-80-26771678/79   Fax: +91-80-26771680   e-mail: bangalore@cbspd.com
- **Chennai:** 20, West Park Road, Shenoy Nagar, Chennai 600 030, Tamil Nadu
  Ph: +91-44-26260666, 26208620   Fax: +91-44-42032115   e-mail: chennai@cbspd.com
- **Kochi:** 36/14 Kalluvilakam, Lissie Hospital Road, Kochi 682 018, Kerala
  Ph: +91-484-4059061-65   Fax: +91-484-4059065   e-mail: cochin@cbspd.com
- **Pune:** Bhuruk Prestige, Sr. No. 52/12/2+1+3/2 Narhe, Haveli
  (Near Katraj-Dehu Road Bypass), Pune 411 041, Maharashtra
  Ph: +91-20-64704058, 64704059, 32342277   Fax: +91-20-24300160   e-mail: pune@cbspd.com

Representatives

•	**Hyderabad**	0-9885175004	•	**Kolkata**	0-9831437309	• **Manipal**	0-9742022075
•	**Mumbai**	0-9833017933	•	**Nagpur**	0-9021734563	• **Patna**	0-9334159340

Printed at Shri Balaji Printer, Delhi - 95

*Dreams are extremely important.
You cannot do it unless you imagine it.*

— **George Lucas**
American film director, producer and screenwriter

By the Same Author

- *Bedside Clinics in Medicine*, Part I (6th edn)
- *Bedside Clinics in Medicine*, Part II (5th edn)
- *Pearls in Medicine for Students* (1st edn)
- A Section on Online Appendix of Kumar and Clark's *Clinical Medicine*, 6th, 7th and 8th (in press) edns
- Chapter in *API Textbook of Medicine*, 8th edn, 2008
- Chapter in *Postgraduate Medicine*, 2009
- Chapters in *Rheumatology: Principles and Practice*, 2010
- Chapters in *Medicine Update* : 2010, 2011 and 2012

Preface to the Fourth Edition

I feel extremely happy and delighted to write the preface of the fourth edition of the book which comes with a new look. The warm welcome accorded to the previous editions has encouraged me to bring out the revised new edition. The book deals with *core knowledge in internal medicine* and follows different *renowned textbooks of medicine* available in the market for the medical students. This volume contains *16 chapters with 2184 questions with single choice answer covering virtually every aspect of medicine* which is required for preparation of different postgraduate medical entrance examinations in the country and abroad.

MCQs are 'windows' through which an aspiring student should peep through, and ultimately give an idea that which part of the 'text' should be read with stress and which not. Deserving students should know that key to success remains in fervent hard work and perseverance. Medicine is a vast science with new horizons being exploded continuously and it is really a tremendous job to read all the pages in voluminous textbooks. Questions are picked up by examiners in a quizzical manner from nooks and corners of unknown pages of huge textbooks and this unpredictability of MCQs forces a student to choose different MCQ books at random, where there is plethora of such books existing in the market and many are yet to come. Success never comes overnight and this is why I think the foundation of medicine should be very strong from the beginning of the preparation; *undergraduate students should be well-conversant with these types of MCQs from the very first day of their clinical training at medical wards.* I am aware that majority likes explanatory answers because students are very comfortable with spoon-feeding and readymade science. I think that no amount of explanation can give success to a student if he/she is not science-bound or text-bound. Very often, the answer changes with a twist in the sequence of questioning resulting in alteration in explanation. As there is no proper guideline for preparation of this type of examinations, students are advised to read these questions dealing with basic medicine meticulously and to get rid of their confusion from standard textbooks. An aspiring student, who refers to textbooks more, hopefully can achieve success in the long run.

My sincere thanks are extended to Mr SK Jain of CBS Publishers for the great care bestowed in publishing the book. No amount of appreciation is sufficient for my family members, my wife Bijoya, daughter Ushasi, and son Abhishek whose active support has helped me in every step to complete the fourth edition.

I convey 'best of luck' to all of my aspiring students.

Arup Kumar Kundu

Preface to the First Edition

Multiple Choice Questions (MCQs) are probably the most sophisticated and widely used component of objective tests to evaluate a student's proficiency and depth of knowledge in a particular subject. MCQs are increasingly used for various entrance examinations where ranking of students is of paramount importance. Unexpected failure may result from lack of familiarity with the MCQ format. This is why I tried to write a book on MCQs dealing with the vast and ever-changing science of medicine for different postgraduate entrance examinations in the country. This volume contains 13 chapters, 1650 questions and covers all major aspects of medicine. All the questions have been arranged systematically. I tried my best to minimize errors by repeated checking. All the questions have their single choice answer present at the bottom of the page for the purpose of quick and easy reading.

It has been observed that questions from the field of medicine cover 15–40% of total bulk of the paper. As questions are asked from every nook and corner of a textbook, it is suggested that students should read the text in between the lines. I hope students will be benefitted in their cut-throat competition of postgraduate entrance examinations like MCI, AIIMS, PGI, BHU, CMC-Vellore, AMU, JIPMER, NIMHANS and different state-controlled examinations, if they pry into it.

I express may sincere thanks to Mr Kaustuv Paul of Crest Infomedia for his constant cooperation in publishing the book. Lastly, I owe my heartfelt gratitude to my family members who assisted me in every step to write the book. Finally, I should say that I will heartily accept sincere suggestions from thoughtful readers.

Arup Kumar Kundu

Contents

Gastroenterology

1. **Parulis is**
   - A. Blue line in the gum in lead poisoning
   - B. Synonymous with Ludwig's angina
   - C. Acute pulpitis
   - D. The pus in the periapical abscess discharging into the oral cavity

2. **Diarrhoea may be associated with all** *except*
   - A. Clindamycin
   - B. Sucralfate
   - C. Digitalis
   - D. Colchicine

3. **Halitosis is present in all** *except*
   - A. Hepatic failure
   - B. Atrophic rhinitis
   - C. Amoebic liver abscess
   - D. Gastrocolic fistula

4. **Passage of a bolus of food through oesophagus is the function of**
   - A. Primary peristaltic wave
   - B. Secondary peristaltic wave
   - C. Tertiary peristaltic wave
   - D. Voluntary phase of deglutition

5. **Oral mucous membrane may be affected in all** *except*
   - A. Stevens-Johnson syndrome
   - B. Pemphigus vulgaris
   - C. Lichen planus
   - D. Dermatitis herpetiformis

6. **Pyrosis is better known as**
   - A. Singultus
   - B. Heartburn
   - C. Water brash
   - D. Retching

7. **Hyperdefaecation is found in all** *except*
   - A. Proctitis
   - B. Irritable bowel syndrome
   - C. Diabetes mellitus
   - D. Hyperthyroidism

8. **Sialorrhoea is associated with all of the following** *except*
   - A. Wilson's disease
   - B. Achalasia cardia
   - C. Carcinoma of the tongue
   - D. Post-encephalitic parkinsonism

Ans: 1-D 2-B 3-C 4-A 5-D 6-B 7-C 8-B

9. **Noma (carcrum oris) may be a feature of all** *except*
   A. Genetic deficiency of catalase
   B. Kala-azar
   C. Measles
   D. Chronic myeloid leukaemia

10. **Aerophagia is commonly found in all** *except*
    A. Rapid eating habit
    B. Hypochondriac personality
    C. Pyloric stenosis
    D. Chronic anxiety states

11. **Macroglossia is not found in**
    A. Bulbar palsy
    B. Primary amyloidosis
    C. Myxoedema
    D. Hurler syndrome

12. **Gum hypertrophy is not a feature of**
    A. Scurvy
    B. Carbamazepine therapy
    C. Acute monocytic leukaemia
    D. Amlodipine therapy

13. **Which statement is true regarding composition of normal stool**
    A. Osmolality 325 mOsm/kg; Na^+16 K^+32 Cl^-40 HCO_3^- 12/litre
    B. Osmolality 400 mOsm/kg; Na^+16 K^+32 Cl^-40 HCO_3^-18/litre
    C. Osmolality 300 mOsm/kg; Na^+40 K^+32 Cl^-16 HCO_3^-40/litre
    D. Osmolality 300 mOsm/kg; Na^+32 K^+75 Cl^-16 HCO_3^-40/litre

14. **Raspberry tongue is found in**
    A. Scarlet fever
    B. Glandular fever
    C. Yellow fever
    D. Rheumatic fever

15. **All of the following are examples of psychiatric illness associated with profound weight loss** *except*
    A. Anorexia nervosa
    B. Schizophrenia
    C. Sheehan's syndrome
    D. Depression

16. **All of the following produce invasive diarrhoea** *except*
    A. *Campylobacter*
    B. *Shigella*
    C. *Clostridium difficile*
    D. *Clostridium perfringens*

17. **Hepatocellular jaundice does not result from**
    A. Rifampicin
    B. Copper sulphate
    C. Halothane
    D. Chlorpropamide

18. **Serum-ascites albumin gradient (SAAG) is > 1.1 g/dl in all** *except*
    A. Tuberculous peritonitis
    B. Congestive cardiac failure
    C. Cirrhosis of liver
    D. Budd-Chiari syndrome

Ans: 9-D 10-C 11-A 12-B 13-D 14-A 15-C 16-D 17-D 18-A

19. All of the following are associated with obstructive jaundice *except*
    A. Oral contraceptives   B. Pregnancy
    C. Crigler-Najjar type II   D. Secondary carcinoma of liver

20. Secretory diarrhoea has no association with
    A. Pancreatic insufficiency
    B. Zollinger-Ellison syndrome
    C. Villous adenoma of rectum
    D. Medullary carcinoma of thyroid

21. WBC in stool is not found in
    A. Giardiasis   B. *Shigella*
    C. *Campylobacter*   D. Entero-invasive *E. coli*

22. Predominant unconjugated hyperbilirubinaemia is defined as
    A. When > 50% of the total serum bilirubin is unconjugated
    B. When > 60% of the total serum bilirubin is unconjugated
    C. When > 70% of the total serum bilirubin is unconjugated
    D. When > 85% of the total serum bilirubin is unconjugated

23. Latent jaundice may be a feature of all *except*
    A. Pernicious anaemia
    B. Acute pulmonary thromboembolism
    C. Tropical sprue
    D. Congestive cardiac failure

24. Which of the following is not a variety of osmotic diarrhoea
    A. Whipple's disease   B. Coeliac disease
    C. Lactase deficiency   D. Laxative abuse

25. Regarding haematochezia, which one is false
    A. Passage of bright red blood per rectum
    B. May be due to rectal polyp, ulcerative colitis or angiodysplasia of colon
    C. The blood may not be mixed with stool
    D. Bleeding source is proximal to ligament of Treitz

26. Which is not a member of familial non-haemolytic hyperbilirubinaemia
    A. Rotor syndrome   B. Reye's syndrome
    C. Dubin-Johnson syndrome   D. Gilbert's syndrome

Ans: 19-C 20-A 21-A 22-D 23-C 24-D 25-D 26-B

27. **Regarding melaena, which statement is false**
    A. At least 60 ml of blood is required
    B. Blood should remain at least 4 hours within the gut
    C. Black tarry semisolid stool
    D. Offensive in odour

28. **Manometric study of lower oesophagus is important in all** *except*
    A. Mallory-Weiss syndrome   B. Polymyositis
    C. Diffuse oesophageal spasm   D. Achalasia cardia

29. **Which one is true in relation to Barrett's oesophagus**
    A. Hiatal hernia may be present in 20% patients
    B. Metaplasia of normal oesophageal squamous epithelium to form columnar epithelium is known as Barrett's oesophagus
    C. A consequence of achalasia cardia
    D. Risk of adenocarcinoma increases 10-fold

30. **Which organ does not move at all with respiration**
    A. Pancreas   B. Transverse colon
    C. Stomach   D. Kidney

31. **Atypical chest pain of reflux oesophagitis is very often precipitated by**
    A. Consumption of food   B. Change of posture
    C. Induction of vomiting   D. Attacks of emotional stress

32. **Achalasia cardia gives rise to all** *except*
    A. Chest pain   B. Heartburn
    C. Dysphagia   D. Regurgitation

33. **Regarding carcinoma of oesophagus, all are true** *except*
    A. Tracheo-oesophageal fistula may occur in advanced disease
    B. Dysphagia starts with solid foods
    C. Odynophagia may be a symptom
    D. Commonest site of affection is lower third

34. **Lower oesophageal sphincter is relaxed by**
    A. Gastrin   B. β-adrenergic agonist
    C. Metoclopramide   D. Protein meal

35. **Carcinoma of oesophagus may be predisposed by all** *except*
    A. Lye ingestion   B. Chronic achalasia cardia
    C. Plummer-Vinson syndrome   D. Hypervitaminosis A

Ans: 27-B 28-A 29-B 30-A 31-B 32-B 33-D 34-B 35-D

36. The water content of adult stool is approximately
    A. 20–30%   B. 40–50%
    C. 50–60%   D. More than 60%

37. Features of Mallory-Weiss syndrome comprise all *except*
    A. Usually involves the lower oesophageal mucosa but also may involve the gastric mucosa near the squamocolumnar junction
    B. May produce melaena
    C. Commonly precipitated by vomiting and retching
    D. In majority of patients, bleeding stops spontaneously

38. Amino acids malabsorption is seen in
    A. Homocystinuria   B. Phenylketonuria
    C. Alkaptonuria   D. Cystinuria

39. Achalasia cardia may lead to all *except*
    A. Pneumonia   B. Lung abscess
    C. Emphysema   D. Fibrosis of the lung

40. Serum alkaline phosphatase is increased in all *except*
    A. Paget's disease of bone   B. Osteomalacia
    C. Sclerosing cholangitis   D. Osteoporosis

41. Regarding *H. pylori*, which statement is false
    A. Gram-negative bacillus
    B. Multiflagellated
    C. It penetrates within the epithelial cells of the stomach
    D. Often resides in the dental plaques of the patient

42. Pyloric stenosis is commonly associated with all *except*
    A. Bilious vomiting
    B. Obliteration of Traube's space tympanicity
    C. Distension of upper abdomen with succussion splash
    D. Visible peristalsis

43. Which statement is false regarding duodenal ulcer
    A. More common in first degree relatives of duodenal ulcer patients
    B. Increased frequency of blood group O and of the non-secretor status
    C. Increased incidence of HLA-B$_5$ antigen
    D. An increase in serum pepsinogen II level

Ans: 36-D 37-A 38-D 39-C 40-D 41-C 42-A 43-D

44. **H. *pylori* is usually not associated with**
    - A. Zollinger-Ellison syndrome B. Antral gastritis
    - C. Non-ulcer dyspepsia D. Gastric lymphoma

45. **The lower oesophageal mucosal ring (Schatzki ring) is**
    - A. A normal oesophageal anatomy
    - B. A cause of haematemesis and/or melaena
    - C. A cause of dysphagia
    - D. A late complication of vagotomy

46. **Regarding diffuse oesophageal spasm, which of the following is true**
    - A. Usually a disease of teen age
    - B. Chest pain mimics angina pectoris
    - C. Invariably requires surgery
    - D. 'Nutcracker' oesophagus is the mildest form

47. **Which of the following does not give rise to haematemesis**
    - A. Carcinoma of the stomach B. Duodenal diverticula
    - C. Mallory-Weiss syndrome D. Stomatostatinoma

48. **The weight of normal daily stool of healthy adult is**
    - A. 100–200 g B. 300–400 g
    - C. 500–600 g D. 700–800 g

49. **NSAID-induced ulcers are best treated by**
    - A. Proton pump inhibitors
    - B. H$_2$-receptor antagonists
    - C. Coating agents like sucralfate
    - D. Prostaglandins like misoprostol

50. **Milk-alkali syndrome (Burnett's syndrome) may lead to all *except***
    - A. Hypercalcaemia
    - B. Hypophosphataemia
    - C. Elevated blood urea nitrogen
    - D. Increased bicarbonate level in serum

51. **All of the following are methods for detection of *H. pylori except***
    - A. Histology B. Endoscopic view
    - C. Polymerase chain reaction D. Rapid urease test

52. **All are absorbed maximally in the upper small intestine *except***
    - A. Folates B. Ca^{++}
    - C. Vitamin B$_{12}$ D. Fe^{++}

Ans: 44-A 45-C 46-B 47-D 48-A 49-D 50-B 51-B 52-C

53. **Treatment of peptic ulcer with magnesium hydroxide is characterised by**
   A. Stronger than H_2-receptor blockers
   B. Suitable for patients with renal impairment
   C. 50% of magnesium is absorbed by the small intestine
   D. Produces loose stool

54. **Acid peptic disease is rarely found in**
   A. Cushing's syndrome
   B. Pregnancy
   C. Polycythaemia vera
   D. Chronic obstructive pulmonary disease

55. **Gastrin is predominantly secreted from**
   A. Antral mucosa   B. Fundus of the stomach
   C. 2nd part of the duodenum   D. Jejunum

56. **Carbenoxolone sodium may be associated with all of the following features** *except*
   A. Development of systemic hypertension
   B. May be associated with milk-alkali syndrome
   C. Complicated by oedema
   D. Development of potassium depletion

57. **Aluminium hydroxide as an antacid may have all characteristics** *except*
   A. Produces constipation
   B. Phosphate depletion is a complication
   C. May lead to Brunner's gland hyperplasia
   D. May contribute to osteomalacia

58. **Late dumping syndrome may be manifested by all** *except*
   A. Diaphoresis   B. Dizziness
   C. Postural hypertension   D. Confusion

59. **The most common gastrointestinal disorder in a community is**
   A. Diverticulitis   B. Duodenal ulcer
   C. Reflux oesophagitis   D. Irritable bowel syndrome

60. **Mallory-Weiss syndrome is commonly seen accompanying**
   A. Reflux oesophagitis   B. Oesophageal carcinoma
   C. Alcoholism   D. Hiatal hernia

Ans: 53-D 54-B 55-A 56-B 57-C 58-C 59-D 60-C

61. **Incidence of stress ulcers in acutely traumatised patients is**
    A. 30–40%   B. 50–60%
    C. 70–80%   D. 90–100%

62. **Which of the following surgical procedures in peptic ulcer most commonly give rise to recurrent ulceration**
    A. Gastroenterostomy
    B. Vagotomy with pyloroplasty
    C. Three-quarter gastric resection
    D. Vagotomy with gastroenterostomy

63. **Regarding cimetidine, all of the following are true** *except*
    A. Related structurally to histamine
    B. May cause mild elevation of serum transaminases and creatinine levels
    C. May produce benign intracranial hypertension
    D. Tender gynaecomastia may be a complication after prolonged use

64. **Silvery stool signifies a lesion characteristic of**
    A. Ileocaecal region   B. Ampulla of Vater
    C. Right colic flexure   D. Meckel's diverticulum

65. **Among the following drugs, which one is thought to be safest in pregnancy**
    A. Sucralfate   B. Misoprostol
    C. Carbenoxolone sodium   D. Omeprazole

66. **All of the following produce hypergastrinaemia** *except*
    A. Lansoprazole therapy   B. Zollinger-Ellison syndrome
    C. Atrophic fundal gastritis   D. Duodenal ulcer

67. **Commonest cause of antral gastritis is**
    A. Alcohol   B. *H. pylori* infection
    C. Pernicious anaemia   D. Herpes virus infection

68. **Chronic gastritis may be characterised by all** *except*
    A. Incessant vomiting   B. Anorexia
    C. Haematemesis   D. Gastric polyp

69. **What percentage of Zollinger-Ellison syndrome are malignant**
    A. 20%   B. 30%
    C. 40%   D. 60%

Ans: 61-D 62-A 63-C 64-B 65-A 66-D 67-B 68-A 69-D

70. All of the following are true in respect to Zollinger-Ellison syndrome *except*
    A. Pancreatic gastrinomas are most common in the head of the pancreas
    B. Solitary primary tumours are very common
    C. Duodenum, hilum of the spleen and rarely the stomach may have gastrinomas
    D. Majority of tumours are biologically malignant

71. The most valuable provocative test of Zollinger-Ellison syndrome is
    A. Feeding of a standard meal B. Calcium infusion test
    C. Secretin injection test   D. Histamine injection test

72. The Zollinger-Ellison syndrome is reported in association with all of the following *except*
    A. Medullary carcinoma of thyroid
    B. Hyperparathyroidism
    C. Phaeochromocytoma
    D. Pituitary adenomas

73. The Zollinger-Ellison syndrome is associated with all of the following *except*
    A. Recalcitrant upper GI ulcers
    B. Diarrhoea and steatorrhoea
    C. Vitamin B_{12} malabsorption
    D. Diagnosis with certainty by BAO/MAO ratio

74. **Chronic afferent loop syndrome producing obstruction may lead to**
    A. Steatorrhoea   B. Hypoglycaemia
    C. Palpitation   D. Recurrent ulceration

75. All of the following endocrine disorders are associated with malabsorption *except*
    A. Diabetes mellitus   B. Adrenal insufficiency
    C. Hyperparathyroidism D. Carcinoid syndrome

76. Chronic gastritis may be associated with all *except*
    A. Gastric atrophy
    B. Intestinal metaplasia
    C. Antibodies to parietal cells
    D. Gastro-oesophageal reflux disease

Ans: 70-B 71-C 72-A 73-D 74-A 75-C 76-D

77. All of the following produce "sub-total villous atrophy' *except*
    A. Radiation   B. Coeliac disease
    C. Hypogammaglobulinaemia D. Abetalipoproteinaemia

78. Upper GI bleeding, angioid streaks in retina and yellowish skin papules indicate
    A. Render-Weber-Osler disease
    B. Ehlers-Danlos syndrome
    C. Pseudoxanthoma elasticum
    D. Peutz-Jeghers syndrome

79. Which of the following has the highest acid secretory effect
    A. Fat   B. Iron
    C. Protein   D. Carbohydrate

80. Menetrier's disease may have all of the following *except*
    A. Large tortuous gastric mucosal folds
    B. Gastritis
    C. Hypoproteinaemia
    D. Hypochlorhydria

81. Extraintestinal amoebiasis may involve all *except*
    A. Skin   B. Heart
    C. Vulva   D. Meninges with encephalon

82. Worldwide, the commonest cause of foreign body obstruction of the GI tract is
    A. Bezoars   B. Enteroliths
    C. Gallstones   D. Parasites

83. In gastroparesis, the following drugs are helpful *except*
    A. Cizapride   B. Tetracycline
    C. Metoclopramide   D. Domperidone

84. All of the following may produce intestinal pseudo-obstruction *except*
    A. Scleroderma   B. Diabetes mellitus
    C. Hyperthyroidism   D. Imipramine

85. Malabsorption may produce all of the following *except*
    A. Cheilosis   B. Achlorhydria
    C. Peripheral neuropathy D. Loss of libido

Ans: 77-D 78-C 79-C 80-B 81-B 82-C 83-B 84-C 85-B

86. A normal faecal fat is defined as
    A. < 6 g for 24 hrs   B. < 9 g for 24 hrs
    C. < 12 g for 24 hrs   D. < 15 g for 24 hrs

87. Which cardiovascular disorder is not associated with steatorrhoea
    A. Constrictive pericarditis
    B. Congestive cardiac failure
    C. Left atrial myxoma
    D. Mesenteric vascular insufficiency

88. All of the following may be associated with diarrhoea *except*
    A. Amitryptiline   B. Colchicine
    C. Sorbitol   D. Theophylline

89. The smallest absorbing unit of the small intestinal mucosa is
    A. Microvillus   B. Crypts
    C. Villus   D. Colummar cells

90. Jejunal diverticula may be associated with
    A. Vitamin B_{12} malabsorption
    B. Hypochlorhydria
    C. Cirrhosis of liver
    D. Chronic pancreatitis

91. Which ion is necessary for active transport of sugars
    A. Calcium   B. Potassium
    C. Magnesium   D. Sodium

92. Fats are ingested primarily in the form of
    A. Monoglycerides   B. Diglycerides
    C. Triglycerides   D. Fatty acids

93. Protein-losing enteropathy may be feature of all *except*
    A. Intestinal tuberculosis   B. Atrial septal defect
    C. Juvenile polyposis coli   D. Chronic cor pulmonale,

94. Tropical sprue may be associated with all *except*
    A. Malabsorption
    B. Patchy lesion
    C. Partial villous atrophy is more common than subtotal villous atrophy
    D. Treatment is done satisfactorily by intestinal resection

Ans: 86-A 87-C 88-A 89-A 90-A 91-D 92-C 93-C 94-D

95. Steatorrhoea accompanying diabetes mellitus may be due to all *except*
    A. Exocrine pancreatic insufficiency
    B. Associated vasculitis
    C. Coexistent coeliac sprue
    D. Abnormal bacterial proliferation in proximal intestine

96. The basic defect in coeliac sprue lies in
    A. Protein metabolism
    B. Fat metabolism
    C. Carbohydrate metabolism
    D. Vitamins and minerals absorption

97. All of the following may give rise to flat oral GTT and a normal IV GTT *except*
    A. Coeliac sprue   B. Whipple's disease
    C. Pancreatic insufficiency   D. Gastric retention

98. All of the following may be associated with hyposplenism *except*
    A. Coeliac disease   B. Haemolytic anaemia
    C. Dermatitis herpetiformis   D. Sickle cell disease

99. Lactose intolerance with lactase deficiency may be present in all *except*
    A. Crohn's disease   B. Giardiasis
    C. Cystic fibrosis   D. Amoebiasis

100. The most reliable screening test in patients suffering from malabsorption is
    A. Quantitative determination of faecal fat
    B. D-xylose absorption test
    C. Radioactive triolein absorption (breath) test
    D. Small intestinal X-rays

101. The most specific treatment in coeliac sprue is
    A. Gluten-free diet   B. Antibiotics
    C. Corticosteroids   D. Folic acid

102. Hepatic amoebiasis is associated with all *except*
    A. May lead to development of amoebic liver abscess
    B. Right lower intercostal tenderness
    C. Abscess commonly affects the right lobe
    D. Jaundice is present in majority

Ans: 95-B 96-A 97-C 98-B 99-D 100-B 101-A 102-D

103. The most common and most specific radiological feature in barium meal follow-through in a patient of malabsorption is
    A. Segmentation and clumping
    B. Coarsening of mucosal folds
    C. Dilatation
    D. Loss of mucosal pattern

104. Water is minimally absorbed from
    A. Caecum
    B. Ascending colon
    C. Transverse colon
    D. Descending colon

105. If intestinal biopsy is not possible, the diagnosis of Whipple's disease can be made by
    A. Lymph node biopsy
    B. Stomach biopsy
    C. Liver biopsy
    D. Rectal biopsy

106. A patient of severe malabsorption having fever, hepato-splenomegaly, lymphadenopathy, sacroiliitis and increased skin pigmentation is probably suffering from
    A. Intestinal lymphoma
    B. Carcinoid syndrome
    C. Whipple's disease
    D. Intestinal lymphangiectasia

107. Treatment of choice in correcting anaemia of "blind loop syndrome' is
    A. Iron
    B. Broad-spectrum antibiotics
    C. Vitamin
    D. Folic acid

108. The major site of bile salt absorption is
    A. Stomach
    B. Duodenum
    C. Proximal small intestine
    D. Distal small intestine

109. Giardiasis is characterised by all except
    A. Infection usually occurs by ingesting contaminated water containing the flagellate form
    B. Malabsorption
    C. Inflammation of duodenal and jejunal mucosa
    D. Lactose intolerance

110. All of the following enzymes may be normally found in stool except
    A. Amylase
    B. Lipase
    C. Pepsin
    D. Trypsin

Ans: 103-C 104-D 105-A 106-C 107-B 108-D 109-A 110-C

111. **All are recognised complications of inflammatory bowel disease** *except*
    A. Gallstone formation   B. Pyoderma gangrenosum
    C. Aphthous stomatitis   D. Erythema marginatum

112. **Intestinal lymphangiectasia is characterised by all** *except*
    A. Hypoproteinaemia and oedema
    B. Low level of transferrin and caeruloplasmin
    C. Malabsorption
    D. Lymphocytosis

113. **Regarding ulcerative colitis, which is true**
    A. Segmental involvement is common
    B. Granuloma and fistula formation are characteristic
    C. Crypt abscesses are typical
    D. Malignancy never follows even in long-standing disease

114. **The inheritance of cystic fibrosis is**
    A. Sex-linked recessive   B. Autosomal recessive
    C. Sex-linked dominant   D. Autosomal dominant

115. **Pseudomembranous colitis is best treated by**
    A. Vancomycin   B. Clindamycin
    C. Tobramycin   D. Erythromycin

116. **Which segment of the GI tract is most susceptible to volvulus**
    A. Caecum   B. Sigmoid colon
    C. Small intestine   D. Stomach

117. **Commonest cause of anaemia after peptic ulcer surgery is**
    A. Iron deficiency   B. Haemolysis
    D. Folic acid deficiency C. Vitamin B_{12} deficiency

118. **Crohn's disease may be complicated by all** *except*
    A. Hydroureter   B. Clubbing
    C. Amyloidosis   D. Chronic cholecystitis

119. **Jejunoileal bypass surgery done for obesity may be complicated by all** *except*
    A. Arthritis   B. Electrolyte imbalance
    C. Emphysema   D. Nephrolithiasis

Ans: 111-D 112-D 113-C 114-B 115-A 116-B 117-A 118-D 119-C

120. *Giardia lamblia* infestation produces a syndrome mimicking
   A. Peptic ulcer disease   B. Irritable bowel syndrome
   C. Tropical sprue   D. Biliary dyspepsia

121. Most helpful differentiating point between ulcerative colitis and Crohn's disease by rectal biopsy is
   A. Granuloma   B. Crypt abscess
   C. Fibrosis   D. Transmural involvement

122. Pyloric stenosis may be complicated by
   A. Acidosis   B. Hyperkalaemia
   C. Hyperchloraemia   D. Hypochloraemic alkalosis

123. 'String sign' in Crohn's disease is due to
   A. Fistula   B. Spasm
   C. Pseudopolyps   D. Small ulceration

124. The commonest manifestation of radiation proctitis is
   A. Diarrhoea   B. Mucous discharge
   C. Pruritus ani   D. Bleeding per rectum

125. All of the following are true regarding Whipple's disease *except*
   A. Gram-negative bacilli *Clostridium whipplei* is responsible
   B. Coronary arteritis may be a feature
   C. Cranial nerve palsy may occur
   D. Commonly manifested by diarrhoea, weight loss with hepato-splenomegaly

126. The causative agent of tropical sprue is
   A. *Shigella*   B. *Campylobacter*
   C. *Yersinia*   D. Unknown

127. Which segment of colon is commonly affected by vascular insufficiency
   A. Ascending colon   B. Hepatic flexure
   C. Transverse colon   D. Splenic flexure

128. Regarding Meckel's diverticulum, which one is false
   A. Present in 2% population
   B. Usually 5 cm long
   C. Present within 100 cm of the ileocaecal valve
   D. May contain oesophageal or rectal mucosa

Ans: 120-B 121-A 122-D 123-B 124-D 125-A 126-D 127-D 128-D

129. **Peritonitis may be complicated by all** *except*
   A. Renal failure
   B. Acute lung injury
   C. Pelvic abscess
   D. Haemorrhagic pancreatitis

130. **Which is true in respect to irritable bowel syndrome**
   A. Most common GI disorder in practice
   B. Commonly affects middle-aged males
   C. Easily treatable
   D. Nocturnal diarrhoea is common

131. **Features of gastric outlet obstruction produced by congenital hypertrophic pyloric stenosis develop in infants**
   A. At birth
   B. Within first 24 hours of birth
   C. During the first 10 days of life
   D. Over the first 4–6 weeks of life

132. **Hirschsprung's disease is not manifested by**
   A. Distended abdomen
   B. Vomiting
   C. Obstipation
   D. Rectal ampulla is full of faeces while the anal sphincter is normal

133. **Commonest complaint by a patient in carcinoma of the rectum is**
   A. Constipation
   B. Pain abdomen
   C. Haematochezia
   D. Anal pain

134. **All of the following are true regarding acute mesenteric vascular occlusion** *except*
   A. Young women are the main victims
   B. Severe periumbilical pain at the onset
   C. Abdominal distension with normal peristaltic sound, even in the face of severe infarction
   D. Barium study of the small intestine reveals 'thumbprinting'

135. **All of the following are true in irritable bowel syndrome** *except*
   A. Usually have 3 clinical components: spastic, diarrhoeal and both
   B. Altered intestinal motility and increased visceral perception are the main pathophysiologic abnormalities
   C. Rectal ampulla is empty but tender sigmoid is full of faeces
   D. Sigmoidoscopy shows multiple small discrete ulcers often covered with slough

---

Ans: 129-D 130-A 131-D 132-D 133-C 134-A 135-D

136. **Crohn's disease may produce all of the following** *except*
    A. Vesicovaginal fistula   B. Rectovesical fistula
    C. Perianal fistula   D. Jejunocolic fistula

137. **Commonest extraintestinal complication of ulcerative colitis is**
    A. Sclerosing cholangitis   B. Arthritis
    C. Pyoderma gangrenosum   D. Uveitis

138. **Symptoms in carcinoma of the left colon include all** *except*
    A. Cramps in the abdomen   B. Melaena
    C. Low back pain   D. Alteration of bowel habit

139. **Which is true regarding irritable bowel syndrome**
    A. Pain abdomen usually lasts for 1/2 hour
    B. Temporary relief of pain by passage of flatus or stool
    C. Nocturnal pain abdomen is frequent complaint
    D. Periodicity is common

140. **Which part of the colonic carcinoma is very easily overlooked**
    A. Hepatic flexure   B. Caecum
    C. Splenic flexure   D. Transverse colon

141. **Crohn's disease is caused by**
    A. Nutritional deficiency
    B. Toxin elaborated by infectious microorganisms
    C. Autoimmunity
    D. Not known

142. **Ulcerative colitis involves the rectal mucosa in**
    A. 30–40%   B. 50–60%
    C. 70–80%   D. 90–100%

143. **Pneumaturia is an established feature of**
    A. Irritable bowel syndrome   B. Intestinal lymphoma
    C. Crohn's disease   D. Coeliac disease

144. **Regarding ischaemic colitis, which one is true**
    A. Affects young population
    B. Almost always an occlusive disease of mesenteric vessels
    C. Rectal bleeding is a rare complication
    D. Angiography is not helpful

Ans: 136-A 137-B 138-B 139-B 140-B 141-D 142-D 143-C 144-D

145. **The commonest small-bowel malignancy is**
    A. Periampullary carcinoma   B. Lymphomas
    C. Adenocarcinomas   D. Leiomyosarcomas

146. **Regarding angiodysplasia of colon, which one is false**
    A. Left colon is commonly affected
    B. Haemotochezia is common
    C. Aortic stenosis may be associated with
    D. It looks like spider angiomas of the skin

147. **Gardner's syndrome may be associated with all** *except*
    A. Fibromas   B. Osteomas
    C. Epidermoid cyst   D. Astrocytoma

148. **Which one is false regarding irritable bowel syndrome**
    A. Sense of complete evacuation
    B. Abdominal distension
    C. Colicky pain abdomen
    D. Mucous diarrhoea or pencil-like pasty stools

149. **Malignant potential is least in**
    A. Villous adenoma of colon   B. Peutz-Jeghers syndrome
    C. Ulcerative colitis   D. Familial colonic polyposis

150. **All of the following are true regarding diverticulitis** *except*
    A. Males are affected more than females
    B. Right side of colon is less affected than the left
    C. Perforation is a serious complication
    D. Massive rectal bleeding is very common

151. **The commonest cause of metastasis to the wall of the stomach is**
    A. Carcinoma of thyroid   B. Carcinoma of breast
    C. Melanoma   D. Hepatoma

152. **All of the following are true regarding right-sided colonic carcinoma** *except*
    A. Cachexia   B. Anaemia
    C. Pain abdomen   D. Alteration of bowel habit

153. **Gastric diverticula are**
    A. Commonly seen
    B. Clinically not significant
    C. Need immediate upper GI endoscopy
    D. A premalignant condition

Ans: 145-A 146-A 147-D 148-A 149-B 150-D 151-C 152-D 153-B

154. Which of the following agent's absorption is least affected in massive small bowel resection
    A. Vitamin B_{12} B. Salt and water
    C. Ca^{++} C. Fat

155. Which of the following is false regarding acute appendicitis
    A. Anorexia is rare
    B. Nausea and vomiting occurs in 50–60% cases
    C. The temperature is usually normal or slightly elevated
    D. Meckel's diverticulitis is one of the close differential diagnosis

156. Which of the following immunoglobulins may be depressed in *Giardia lamblia* infestation
    A. IgG   B. IgA
    C. IgM   D. IgD

157. Which of the following may develop into intestinal lymphoma
    A. Coeliac disease   B. Ulcerative colitis
    C. Eosinophilic enteritis   D. Intestinal lymphangiectasia

158. The maximum absorption of fluid in the gastrointestinal tract occurs in
    A. Stomach   B. Jejunum
    C. Ileum   D. Colon

159. Melanosis coli indicates
    A. Anthraquinone laxative abuse
    B. Hypereosinophilic enteritis
    C. Crohn's disease
    D. Melanoma affecting colon

160. Which of the following is not responsible for food poisoning
    A. *Bacillus cereus*   B. *Clostridium botulinum*
    C. *Streptococcus* (Gr. A)   D. *Clostridium perfringens*

161. All of the following may cause traveller's diarrhoea *except*
    A. Enterotoxigenic *E. coli*   B. *Campylobacter jejuni*
    C. Rota and norwalk viruses   D. *Clostridium difficile*

162. All are major components of intestinal gas *except*
    A. CO_2 B. N_2
    C. H_2S D. Methane

Ans: 154-B 155-A 156-B 157-A 158-B 159-A 160-C 161-D 162-C

163. **Among all of the following, which is the most characteristic feature regarding intestinal ischaemia**

    A. Fever
    B. Sinus tachycardia
    C. Discordance between subjective symptoms and objective findings
    D. Bloody diarrhoea

164. **All of the following protozoal infections produce diarrhoea in a patient of AIDS** *except*

    A. *Isospora belli*
    B. Microsporidia
    C. *Cryptosporidium*
    D. *Mycobacterium avium-intracellulare*

165. **Which of the following is false regarding cholera**

    A. Onset with purging
    B. Offensive stool
    C. Absence of tenesmus
    D. Subnormal surface temperature

166. **In coeliac sprue, which of the following is non-deficient in the body**

    A. Vitamin B_{12} B. Folic acid
    C. Iron   D. Serum albumin

167. **Hour-glass stomach is usually produced by**

    A. Lymphoma   B. Syphilis
    D. Developmental anomaly   D. Gastric ulcer

168. **Bacillary dysentery can be differentiated from ulcerative colitis by**

    A. Barium enema   B. Stool culture
    C. Stool smear   D. Sigmoidoscopy

169. **Commonest site of carcinoma of the stomach is**

    A. Prepyloric
    B. Lesser curvature
    C. Greater curvature
    D. Body of the stomach

170. **Which of the following is not included in the list of high-folate diet**

    A. Vegetables   B. Liver
    C. Milk   D. Fruits

Ans: 163-C 164-D 165-B 166-B 167-D 168-B 169-A 170-C

171. **Commonest type of oral malignancy is**
    A. Adenocarcinoma
    B. Basal cell carcinoma
    C. Melanoma
    D. Squamous cell carcinoma

172. **Severe mucoid diarrhoea which is rich in electrolytes should arouse suspicion of**
    A. Carcinoid syndrome
    B. Villous adenoma of the colon
    C. Zollinger-Ellison syndrome
    D. Irritable bowel syndrome

173. **Burst abdomen commonly occurs on the**
    A. 1st day
    B. 2nd day
    C. 3rd day
    D. 7th day

174. **Which one of the following is not an ocular complication of ulcerative colitis**
    A. Uveitis
    B. Cataract
    C. Scleromalacia perforans
    D. Episcleritis

175. **Commonest cause of colonic obstruction is**
    A. Hernia
    B. Volvulus
    C. Neoplasm
    D. Adhesions

176. **Commonest site of carcinoid tumour is**
    A. Stomach
    B. Ileum
    C. Appendix
    D. Colon

177. **Which site of gastric carcinoma is easily overlooked by barium meal study**
    A. Cardia
    B. Lesser curvature
    C. Body
    D. Antrum

178. **One of the earliest manifestations of cystic fibrosis is**
    A. Gram-negative sepsis
    B. Malabsorption
    C. Meconium ileus
    D. Tetany

179. **The ideal time to give antacids in peptic ulcer disease is**
    A. Just before meals
    B. Immediately after meals
    C. One hour after meals and at bedtime
    D. With the meals

Ans: 171-D 172-B 173-D 174-B 175-C 176-C 177-A 178-C 179-C

180. Which endocrine disorder is associated with exudative ascites
    A. Conn's syndrome
    B. Addison's disease
    C. Hyperparathyroidism
    D. Hypothyroidism

181. The single most important point which differentiates tropical sprue from coeliac sprue is
    A. Type of anaemia
    B. Small intestinal biopsy
    C. D-xylose absorption test
    D. Response to treatment

182. Major organ for the removal of gastrin is
    A. Liver
    B. Lung
    C. Kidney
    D. Intestine

183. Desire for defaecation is initiated by
    A. Distention of the sigmoid colon
    B. Contraction of the rectum
    C. Distention of the rectum
    D. Contraction of the internal anal sphincter

184. Commonest cause of upper GI bleeding in an alcoholic is
    A. Acute gastritis
    B. Ruptured oesophageal varices
    C. Mallory-Weiss syndrome
    D. Duodenal ulcer

185. Presence of diverticulosis is most commonly seen in
    A. Transverse colon
    B. Sigmoid colon
    C. Descending colon
    D. Caecum

186. Diabetic diarrhoea may be encountered in the presence of
    A. Nephropathy
    B. Neuropathy
    C. Retinopathy
    D. Macroangiopathy

187. Which of the following primaries is uncommonly associated with bony metastasis
    A. Thyroid
    B. Colon
    C. Breast
    D. Prostate

188. Characteristics of anorexia nervosa include all *except*
    A. Hypothermia
    B. Amenorrhoea
    C. Carotenaemia
    D. Loss of axillary and pubic hair

Ans: 180-D 181-D 182-C 183-C 184-A 185-B 186-B 187-B 188-B

189. Which of the following is not effective to eradicate *H. pylori*
    A. Clarithromycin
    C. Tinidazole
    B. Pantoprazole
    D. Cefixime

190. Commonest cause of duodenal haematoma is
    A. Haemophilia
    D. Acute leukaemia
    B. Anticoagulant therapy
    D. Trauma

191. Carcinoid syndrome
    A. Is multiple in 1/5th cases
    D. More common in women
    B. Produces jaundice
    C. Increases BP

192. Incidence of gastric carcinoid is increased in all *except*
    A. Achlorhydria
    C. Mesenteric fibrosis
    B. Hashimoto's thyroiditis
    D. Pernicious anaemia

193. Which of the following is false regarding pernicious anaemia
    A. 90% have anti-parietal cell antibody
    B. Gastric polyp is common
    C. 60% have anti-intrinsic factor antibody
    D. It is a common cause of haemolytic anaemia in the West

194. All the drugs are given sometime in the treatment of carcinoid syndrome *except*
    A. β-adrenergic agonist
    B. $H_1 + H_2$ receptor antagonist
    C. Serotonin antagonist
    D. Methylxanthine bronchodilators

195. Which of the following infections may produce features like cardiospasm
    A. Schistosomiasis
    C. Trichinosis
    B. Trypanosomiasis
    D. Leishmaniasis

196. Most reliable method of measuring steatorrhoea is
    A. Schilling test
    C. Faecal fat estimation
    B. D-xylose absorption test
    D. Small intestinal mucosal biopsy

197. Geographic tongue is ideally treated by
    A. Vitamin B-complex
    C. Folic acid
    B. Iron
    D. None of the above

198. Carcinoma of the large intestine is mostly found in
    A. Caecum
    C. Transverse colon
    B. Sigmoid colon
    D. Ascending colon

Ans: 189-D 190-D 191-A 192-C 193-D 194-A 195-B 196-C 197-D 198-B

199. **Whipple's triad is found in**
    A. Somatostatinoma   B. Insulinoma
    C. Carcinoid syndrome   D. Glucagonoma

200. **Botulism may be associated with all of the following** *except*
    A. Diplopia   B. Constipation
    C. Increased salivation   D. Descending paralysis

201. **Gluten-free diet is beneficial in**
    A. Dermatitis herpetiformis B. Atopic eczema
    C. Psoriasis   D. Pemphigus

202. **Pseudomembranous colitis is not produced by**
    A. Chloramphenicol   B. Ampicillin
    C. Clindamycin   D. Streptomycin

203. **Normally in health, the venous flow in abdominal superficial veins is**
    A. Towards the umbilicus   B. From below upwards
    C. Away from the umbilicus D. From above downwards

204. **Anti-LKM$_1$ antibodies (liver–kidney microsomes) are seen in infection with**
    A. Hepatitis B   B. Hepatitis C
    C. Hepatitis D   D. Cytomegalovirus

205. **Which of the following is not a disorder of intestinal motility**
    A. Irritable bowel syndrome B. Intestinal pseudo-obstruction
    C. Ulcerative colitis   D. Diverticulosis

206. **The novel agent tegaserod is used in**
    A. Ulcerative colitis
    B. Irritable bowel syndrome
    C. Coeliac disease
    D. Gastro-oesophageal reflux disease

207. **Mucosal immunity is mainly due to**
    A. IgG   B. IgA
    D. IgM   D. IgD

208. **A child having diarrhoea later complicated by appearance of rash and petechiae. The most probable diagnosis is**
    A. *Campylobacter*   B. *Shigella*
    C. *Yersinia*   D. Rota virus

Ans: 199-B 200-C 201-A 202-D 203-C 204-B 205-C 206-B 207-B 208-B

209. **A 'white patch' in the throat may be due to all** *except*
   A. Ludwig's angina
   B. Diphtheria
   C. Infectious mononucleosis
   D. Streptococcal infection

210. **Gluten-induced enteropathy is strongly associated with**
   A. HLA-DQ$_1$
   B. HLA-DR$_4$
   C. HLA-DR$_3$
   D. HLA-B$_8$

211. **Which vitamin deficiency is commonly seen in Crohn's disease**
   A. Vitamin A
   B. Vitamin D
   C. Folic acid
   D. Vitamin B$_{12}$

212. **Which is true in familial polyposis coli**
   A. X-linked recessive inheritance
   B. The rectum is spared
   C. The patient may not have any symptom until a carcinoma has developed
   D. Polyps are present since birth

213. **Michaelis-Gutmann bodies are found in**
   A. Pneumatosis cystoides intestinalis
   B. Malakoplakia of colon
   C. Pseudomyxoma peritonei
   D. Diverticulosis of colon

214. **Anti-saccharomyces cerevisiae antibody (ASCA) is classically present in**
   A. Primary sclerosing cholangitis
   B. Crescentic glomerulonephritis
   C. Wegener's granulomatosis
   D. Ulcerative colitis

215. **Saint's triad is presence of gallstones, hiatal hernia and**
   A. Diverticulosis
   B. Pancreatitis
   C. Haemorrhoids
   D. Gastro-oesophageal reflux disease

216. **Hyperdefaecation is characteristic of all** *except*
   A. Irritable bowel syndrome
   B. Diverticulitis
   C. Hyperthyroidism
   D. Proctitis

Ans: 209-A 210-C 211-D 212-C 213-B 214-D 215-A 216-B

217. **Faecal assay of α_1-antitrypsin clinches the diagnosis of**
    A. Cirrhosis of liver
    B. Irritable bowel syndrome
    C. Protein-losing enteropathy
    D. Chronic pancreatitis

218. **Typhlitis may be associated with all *except***
    A. Responds to medical treatment
    B. Common in neutropenic patients in acute leukaemias
    C. Having periumbilical tenderness
    D. Associated with bloody diarrhoea

219. **Among the gastrointestinal peptides, bombesin is**
    A. Peptide yy
    B. Vasoactive intestinal peptide
    C. Neuropeptide y
    D. Gastric inhibitory peptide

220. **Which is true regarding Vincent's angina**
    A. Superficial ulcers in mouth
    B. May be complicated by angina pectoris
    C. Hiatus hernia may be associated with
    D. Gum is the principal site of affection

221. **Large gastric folds are seen in all *except***
    A. Menetrier's disease
    B. Chronic *H. pylori* infection
    C. Sarcoidosis
    D. Gastric malignancy

222. **Barry J Marshall and Robin Warren received Nobel Prize for discovery of *H. pylori* in the year**
    A. 1989   B. 1998
    C. 2003   D. 2005

223. **Constipation may develop from all *except***
    A. Clonidine   B. Cholestyramine
    C. Colchicine   D. Calcium-channel blocker

224. **'Puddle sign' detects small amount of free fluid in peritoneal cavity which may be as low as**
    A. 70 ml   B. 120 ml
    C. 200 ml   D. 270 ml

Ans: 217-C 218-C 219-C 220-D 221-B 222-D 223-C 224-B

225. **Regarding solitary rectal ulcer syndrome (SRUS), which of the following is false**

    A. Commonly in the posterior wall of rectum
    B. Rectal prolapse and straining by patient are common associations
    C. Rectal bleeding and tenesmus are common
    D. Surgery by resection rectopexy may be done

226. **Which of the following is not a recognized complication of ulcerative colitis**

    A. Autoimmune haemolytic anaemia
    B. Pyoderma gangrenosum
    C. Sacroiliitis
    D. Bronchiectasis

227. **Which of the following does not produce secretory diarrhoea**

    A. Hyperparathyroidism
    B. Medullary carcinoma of the thyroid gland
    C. Carcinoid syndrome
    D. Zollinger-Ellison syndrome

Ans: 225-A 226-D 227-A

Hepatobiliary and Pancreatic Disorders

1. Which one of the following originates from non-β islet cell tumour of pancreas
   - A. Insulinoma
   - B. Glucagonoma
   - C. Gastrinoma
   - D. Somatostatinoma

2. Classical triad in carcinoid syndrome is
   - A. Dyspnoea, flushing, valvular heart disease
   - B. Flushing, diarrhoea, valvular heart disease
   - C. Pruritus, wheezing, diarrhoea
   - D. Telangiectasias, flushing, diarrhoea

3. The valvular heart disease common in carcinoid syndrome is
   - A. Mitral stenosis
   - B. Tricuspid incompetence
   - C. Pulmonary incompetence
   - D. Aortic incompetence

4. All are examples of APUDomas *except*
   - A. Melanoma
   - B. Hepatoma
   - C. Phaeochromocytoma
   - D. Medullary carcinoma of thyroid gland

5. Carcinoid syndrome is commonly produced, when the site of primary tumour is present in
   - A. Midgut
   - B. Stomach
   - C. Bronchus
   - D. Hindgut

6. Octreotide can be used in all *except*
   - A. Oesophageal variceal bleeding
   - B. Short bowel syndrome
   - C. Pancreatic ascites
   - D. Ulcerative colitis

Ans: 1-C 2-B 3-B 4-B 5-A 6-D

7. Necrolytic migratory erythema is a feature of
   A. Hepatoblastoma   B. Glucagonoma
   C. Insulinoma   D. Carcinoid syndrome

8. Which of the following is not included in the classical triad of chronic pancreatitis
   A. Diabetes mellitus   B. Abdominal pain
   C. Pancreatic calcification   D. Steatorrhoea

9. Acute pancreatitis may be caused by
   A. Measles   B. Propranolol
   C. *Legionella pneumoniae*   D. Thiazides

10. Elevation in 5-HIAA (hydroxyindoleacetic acid) in urine is found in all *except*
    A. Carcinoid syndrome   B. Coeliac sprue
    C. Whipple's disease   D. Systemic mastocytosis

11. Which of the following pancreatic islet cells synthesizes glucagon
    A. Alpha   B. Beta
    C. Non-beta   D. Delta

12. Which of the following is not a cause of hyperamylasaemia
    A. Renal insufficiency   B. Burns
    C. Acute intermittent prophyria D. Pseudopancreatic cyst

13. Acute pancreatitis may eventually lead to all of the following *except*
    A. Acute lung injury
    B. Fulminant hepatocellular failure
    C. Disseminated intravascular coagulation
    D. Renal failure

14. Bentiromide test diagnoses
    A. Pancreatic ductal obstruction B. Exocrine pancreatic function
    C. Pancreatic carcinoma   D. Endocrine pancreatic function

15. All are recognised complications of acute pancreatitis *except*
    A. Pancreatic phlegmon   B. Pancreatic pseudocyst
    C. Pancreatic ascites   D. Pancreatic malignancy

16. Commonest type of pancreatic carcinoma is
    A. Ductal adenocarcinoma   B. Islet cell carcinoma
    C. Cystadenocarcinoma   D. Mucinous carcinoma

Ans: 7-B 8-B 9-D 10-D 11-A 12-C 13-B 14-B 15-D 16-A

17 Which of the following is false according to Ranson/Imrie criteria in acute pancreatitis for adversely affecting survival on admission

A. Serum LDH > 400 IU/L
B. Serum AST > 400 IU/L
C. Hperglycaemia > 200 mg/dl
D. Leucocytosis > 16000/mm^3

18. Acute pancreatitis is not associated with

A. Hyperparathyroidism   B. Billiary tract disease
C. Pancreatic carcinoma   D. Pancreatic islet cell tumour

19. Endopeptidases include all *except*

A. Trypsin   B. Elastase
C. Chymotrypsin   D. Carboxypeptidase

20. Which of the following clotting factors retains its activity in hepatocellular disorder

A. II   B. VIII
C. IX   D. VII

21. Which one of the following is not a space-occupying disease of liver

A. Gummas   B. Metastatic tumour
C. Amyloid   D. Cyst

22. Commonest cause of pancreatic calcification is

A. Alcohol abuse   B. Protein-energy malnutrition
C. Hyperthyroidism   D. Pancreatic carcinoma

23. Hyperamylasaemia may be caused by all *except*

A. Ruptured ectopic pregnancy B. Administration of morphine
C. Diabetic ketoacidosis   D. Basal pneumonia

24. Which of the following is a predisposing factor for the development of pancreatic carcinoma

A. Cigarette smoking   B. Alcohol abuse
C. Cholelithiasis   D. Macroamylasaemia

25. In exocrine pancreatic insufficiency, which of the following tests remains normal

A. D-xylose absorption test
B. Secretin test
C. Quantitative estimation of faecal fat
D. Bentiromide test

Ans: 17-B 18-D 19-D 20-B 21-C 22-A 23-D 24-A 25-A

26. **Commonest cause of chronic relapsing pancreatitis is**
    A. Trauma
    B. Gallstones
    C. Alcohol abuse
    D. Infection

27. **Venous prominence present at the upper abdomen with direction of flow towards pelvis suggests**
    A. Inferior vena caval obstruction
    B. Portal hypertension
    C. Superior vena caval obstruction
    D. Hepatic vein thrombosis

28. **All of the following produce pancreatic calcification *except***
    A. Hereditary pancreatitis
    B. Alcohol abuse
    C. Protein-energy malnutrition
    D. Insulinoma

29. **Which of the following is not a feature of 'pancreatic cholera'**
    A. Watery diarrhoea
    B. Hypokalaemia
    C. Hypoglycaemia
    D. Hypochlorhydria

30. **The best single diagnostic test for cystic fibrosis is**
    A. Quantitative pilocarpine iontophoresis test
    B. Serum amylase
    C. Serum lipase
    D. Quantitative faecal fat estimation

31. **Which of the following bile acids is virtually absent in advanced cirrhosis of liver**
    A. Deoxycolic acid
    B. Chenodeoxycolic acid
    C. Lithocolic acid
    D. Cholic acid

32. **Zieve's syndrome in alcoholic cirrhosis includes pain abdomen and haemolytic anaemia; the other component is**
    A. Hyperlipidaemia
    B. Hypercalcaemia
    C. Hypergastrinaemia
    D. Hyperamylasaemia

33. **Which of the following is the most sensitive and test of choice in diagnosing cystic duct obstruction, i.e. acute cholecystitis**
    A. Ultrasonography
    B. CT scan
    C. ERCP
    D. HIDA scan

Ans: 26-C 27-C 28-D 29-C 30-A 31-A 32-A 33-D

34. Serum alkaline phosphatase level may be increased in all *except*
    - A. Cholestasis
    - B. Paget's disease
    - C. Metastasis in liver
    - D. Hypervitaminosis D

35. A patient is having isolated elevation of serum alkaline phosphatase. The next test to be performed is
    - A. USG of liver
    - B. δ-glutamyl transpeptidase (CGT) estimation
    - C. Protein electrophoresis
    - D. Bone scan

36. Severe kwashiorkor may have hepatic lesion in the form of
    - A. Fatty infiltration
    - B. Laennec's cirrhosis
    - C. Hepatitis-like picture
    - D. Hepatic vein thrombosis

37. Oral contraceptive pills may have hepatic lesion in the form of all *except*
    - A. Peliosis hepatis
    - B. Hepatic granulomas
    - C. Benign adenomas in liver
    - D. Budd-Chiari syndrome

38. High transaminase level may be found in all *except*
    - A. Acute viral hepatitis
    - B. Chronic pancreatitis
    - C. Right-sided heart failure
    - D. Acute myocardial infarction

39. The major immunoglobulin in primary biliary cirrhosis is
    - A. IgM
    - B. IgA
    - C. IgG
    - D. IgD

40. Which one of the following is false regarding type B hepatitis serology
    - A. Persistence of HBsAg>6 months implies carrier state
    - B. HbeAg implies high infectivity
    - C. Anti-HBs appears to reflect immunity
    - D. IgG anti-HBc indicates acute hepatitis B virus infection

41. Secretin is produced in largest quantities in
    - A. Jejunum
    - B. Stomach
    - C. Duodenum
    - D. Ileum

42. Pruritus associated with cholestasis is mostly seen
    - A. On the palms and soles
    - B. At daytime
    - C. After a cold bath
    - D. In males

Ans: 34-D 35-B 36-A 37-B 38-B 39-A 40-D 41-C 42-A

43. **Which of the following is not associated with leucocytosis**
    A. Toxic hepatitis B. Acute viral hepatitis
    C. Weil's disease D. Amoebic liver abscess

44. **Hepatic rub may be found in**
    A. Haemangioma of liver B. Hepatic neoplasm
    C. Acute viral hepatitis D. Pyogenic liver abscess

45. **Vitamin K absorption is dependent on**
    A. HCl B. Bile salts
    C. Bilirubin D. Succus entericus

46. **The best way to diagnose Gilbert's syndrome is**
    A. Testing for red blood cell survival
    B. Liver biopsy
    C. Bromsulphalein (BSP) excretion test
    D. 48 hours fasting with only 300 cal/day

47. **Differential diagnosis of jaundice includes all** *except*
    A. Argyria B. Carotenaemia
    C. Atabrine toxicity D. Diffuse xanthomatosis

48. **The presence of hepatic bruit over the liver suggests**
    A. Recent liver biopsy B. Perihepatitis
    C. Hepatoma D. Portal hypertension

49. **Predominant unconjugated hyperbilirubinaemia is seen in all** *except*
    A. Shunt hyperbilirubinaemia B. Dubin-Johnson syndrome
    C. Gilbert's syndrome D. Crigler-Najjar syndrome

50. **Cholestasis is the retention of all substances in the blood** *except*
    A. Triglycerides B. Bile salts
    C. Vitamin D D. Cholesterol

51. **Bedside diagnosis of obstructive jaundice includes all** *except*
    A. Generalised pruritus B. Palpable gallbladder
    C. High-coloured stool D. Xanthelasma

52. **Characteristic of hepatic pre-coma is**
    A. Night-time somnolence B. Flaccid muscles
    C. Babinski's sign D. Presence of ankle clonus

Ans: 43-B 44-B 45-B 46-D 47-A 48-C 49-B 50-C 51-C 52-D

53. **Leptospirosis can be diagnosed during the 1st week of illness by**
    A. Urine analysis
    B. Stool culture
    C. Dark-field examination
    D. Agglutination test

54. **All of the following are present in hepatic coma *except***
    A. Asterixis
    B. Abnormal EEC
    C. Absent deep reflexes
    D. Increased ammonia level in blood

55. **Commonest form of hepatic tuberculosis is**
    A. Miliary tuberculosis
    B. Tuberculomas
    C. Tuberculous hepatitis
    D. Tuberculous abscess

56. **The earliest and most common metabolic abnormality in hepatic encephalopathy is**
    A. Respiratory alkalosis
    B. Metabolic alkalosis
    C. Respiratory acidosis
    D. Metabolic acidosis

57. **Which of the following surgeries is related to severe hepatocellular dysfunction**
    A. Vagotomy
    B. Jejunoileal bypass
    C. Pyloroplasty
    D. Gastric bypass

58. **Which of the following clotting factors is not produced in the liver**
    A. II
    B. VII
    C. IV
    D. V

59. **Which of the following drugs is not associated with cholestasis**
    A. Erythromycin stearate
    B. Chlorpropamide
    C. Chlorpromazine
    D. Methyl testosterone

60. **Which of the following infections commonly produces hepatic granuloma**
    A. *Pneumococcus*
    B. *Leptospira*
    C. *Brucella abortus*
    D. LD body

61. **Which is not true so far as definition of cirrhosis of liver is concerned**
    A. Fatty infiltration
    B. Necrosis
    C. Fibrosis
    D. Regeneration

Ans: 53-C 54-A 55-A 56-A 57-B 58-C 59-A 60-C 61-A

62. **What is true about Weil's disease**
    A. Low glucose in CSF
    B. Leucopenia
    C. Liver biopsy is diagnostic
    D. Myocarditis may be a complication

63. **Spider naevi**
    A. Are pathognomonic of portal hypertension
    B. May be seen in some healthy people
    C. Often seen in first trimester of pregnancy
    D. Correlates with the amount of urinary oestradiol excretion

64. **Chronic active hepatitis may have all the following features** *except*
    A. Amenorrhoea   B. Arthralgia
    C. Jaundice   D. Haematemesis

65. **Following cardiac surgery of which valve operation is most likely
    to develop jaundice**
    A. Mitral valve   B. Tricuspid valve
    C. Aortic valve   D. Pulmonary valve

66. **Among the undermentioned liver function tests, which one is least
    likely to be impaired during normal pregnancy**
    A. Serum albumin   B. Serum transaminases
    C. Serum cholesterol   D. Serum bilirubin

67. **Congenital hepatic fibrosis may be associated with**
    A. Atrial septal defect
    B. Medullary sponge kidney
    C. Retroperitoneal fibrosis
    D. Endocardial fibroelastosis

68. **Which is true in halothane-induced hepatitis**
    A. Males are commonly susceptible
    B. Splenomegaly
    C. Marked cholestasis
    D. Peripheral eosinophilia

69. **The prostaglandins are**
    A. Proteins   B. Enzymes
    C. Polysaccharides   D. Fatty acids

Ans: 62-D 63-B 64-D 65-A 66-B 67-B 68-D 69-D

70. **Hyperbilirubinaemia is not associated with**
    A. Hereditary spherocytosis
    B. Pulmonary alveolar proteinosis
    C. Budd-Chiari syndrome
    D. Dubin-Johnson syndrome

71. **Which light source produces best photodecomposition of bilirubin**
    A. Ultraviolet   B. Fluorescent
    C. Sunlight   D. Moonlight

72. **The most sensitive test which detects hepatic involvement in congestive cardiac failure is**
    A. Level of transaminases
    B. Serum bilirubin assay
    C. Bromsulphalein (BSP) excretion test
    D. Serum albumin estimation

73. **The principal lipid contents of human bile are all *except***
    A. Free fatty acids   B. Conjugated bile salts
    C. Cholesterol   D. Lecithin

74. **Fatty liver may be produced by**
    A. Chloramphenicol   B. Oral contraceptives
    C. Anabolic steroids   D. Tetracycline

75. **Commonest micro-organism responsible for cholangitis is**
    A. *E. coli*   B. *Klebsiella pneumoniae*
    C. *Streptococcus faecalis* D. *Salmonella*

76. **Commonest malignant tumour of gallbladder is**
    A. Squamous cell carcinoma   B. Adenocarcinoma
    C. Haemangioendothelioma   D. Sarcoma

77. **Cholangiocarcinoma may be associated with**
    A. Cholelithiasis   B. Ulcerative colitis
    C. *Tinea echinococcus* infestation D. Biliary atresia

78. **Reye's syndrome may be associated with all *except***
    A. Moderate jaundice
    B. Elevated aminotransferases
    C. Hypoglycaemia
    D. Chickenpox as a precipitating factor

Ans: 70-B 71-B 72-C 73-A 74-D 75-A 76-B 77-B 78-A

79. **Which is true regarding rapidly shrinking liver in fulminant hepatic failure**
    A. The disease process is improving
    B. A fluctuating clinical course
    C. A bad prognosis
    D. Means nothing to clinical course

80. **In complete biliary obstruction, urinary urobilinogen is**
    A. Decreased
    B. Elevated
    C. Remains normal
    D. Episodic increase and decrease

81. **Which is false regarding Reye's syndrome**
    A. Mitochondrial dysfunction of liver
    B. Salicylates may be responsible
    C. There may be cerebral oedema
    D. Survivors pass on to chronic liver disease

82. **All are recognised complications of acute viral hepatitis** *except*
    A. Polyarteritis nodosa   B. Aplastic anaemia
    C. Meningitis   D. Myocarditis

83. **Serum-ascites albumin gradient (SAAG) is > 1.1 g/dl in all** *except*
    A. Nephrotic syndrome   B. Congestive cardiac failure
    C. Portal hypertension   D. Fulminant hepatic failure

84. **All of the following may be associated with hypoglobulinaemia** *except*
    A. Severe combined immunodeficiency
    B. AIDS
    C. Multiple myeloma
    D. Chronic lymphatic leukaemia

85. **All of the following are features of hepatocellular failure** *except*
    A. Fetor hepaticus   B. Ascites
    C. Flapping tremor   D. Haematemesis

86. **All are associated with low serum caeruloplasmin level** *except*
    A. Newborn and infants (up to 6 months)
    B. Protein-losing enteropathies
    C. Wilson's disease
    D. Polycystic kidney disease

Ans: 79-C 80-A 81-D 82-C 83-A 84-B 85-D 86-D

87. **All of the following may be the aetiology of Budd-Chiari syndrome** *except*

    A. Congenital hepatic fibrosis
    B. Antiphospholipid syndrome
    C. Oral contraceptive pills
    D. Right atrial myxoma

88. **Serum of patient contains only anti-HBs; he is**

    A. Acutely infected by type B virus
    B. Suffering from chronic hepatitis B virus infection
    C. Low level of HbsAg carrier
    D. Vaccinated

89. **All of the following may produce hepatic granuloma** *except*

    A. Losartan   B. INH
    C. Allopurinol   D. Sulphonamides

90. **Minimal free fluid in the abdomen required to be diagnosed by ultrasonography is**

    A. 15 ml   B. 30 ml
    C. 75 ml   D. 100 ml

91. **Which one of the following is false in hepatorenal syndrome**

    A. Slow-onset azotaemia in chronic liver disease
    B. Urine Na$^+$ concentration >10 mEq/dl
    C. Urine to plasma osmolality ratio >1.0
    D. Urine to plasma creatinine ratio >30

92. **Which one of the following is false in mesenteric cyst**

    A. Moves freely at right angles to the line of attachment of the mesentery
    B. A well-defined cystic swelling in abdomen
    C. Positive 'puddle sign'
    D. Positive fluid thrill

93. **Non-cirrhotic portal fibrosis may be associated with**

    A. Oral contraceptives   B. Chronic arsenic ingestion
    C. Sarcoidosis   D. Umbilical sepsis

94. **All are causes of chylous ascites** *except*

    A. Intra-abdominal malignancy
    B. Thrombosis of mesenteric artery
    C. Tuberculosis
    D. Filariasis

Ans: 87-A 88-D 89-A 90-B 91-B 92-C 93-B 94-B

95. **Primary biliary cirrhosis may be associated with all** *except*
    A. Wilson's disease
    B. CREST syndrome
    C. Renal tubular acidosis
    D. Autoimmune thyroiditis

96. **Minimal fluid required to have classical shifting dullness in ascites is**
    A. 100–250 ml
    B. 250–500 ml
    C. 500–1000 ml
    D. More than 1 litre

97. **Hepatitis-like feature may be seen in therapy with all** *except*
    A. Atorvastatin
    B. Ketoconazole
    C. INH
    D. Zidovudine

98. **Example of transudative ascites is**
    A. Malignant peritonitis
    B. Budd-Chiari syndrome
    C. Cirrhosis of liver
    D. Chylous ascites

99. **Chronicity in hepatitis C virus infection is**
    A. 10%
    B. 30%
    C. 50%
    D. 80%

100. **In gallbladder disease, plain abdominal X-ray may diagnose all** *except*
    A. Limey bile
    B. Acalculous cholecystitis
    C. Porcelain gallbladder
    D. Emphysematous cholecystitis

101. **All of the following may present as latent jaundice** *except*
    A. Pernicious anaemia
    B. Acute pancreatitis
    C. Pyloric stenosis
    D. Acute myocardial infarction

102. **Acalculous cholecystitis may be precipitated by all** *except*
    A. Vasculitis
    B. Torsion of the gallbladder
    C. Diabetes mellitus
    D. Cholelithiasis

103. **Normal portal venous pressure is**
    A. < 5 mm Hg
    B. >12 mm Hg
    C. 5–7 mm Hg
    D. 7–10 mm Hg

104. **Endoscopic retrograde cholagiopancreatography (ERCP) has all the advantages** *except*
    A. Best visualisation of cystic duct
    B. Endoscopic sphincterotomy and stone removal
    C. Biliary manometry
    D. Bile or pancreatic cytology

Ans: 95-A 96-C 97-A 98-C 99-C 100-B 101-C 102-D 103-C 104-A

105. **All of the following produce deep jaundice** *except*
   A. G6PD deficiency
   B. Recurrent cholestasis of pregnancy
   C. Carcinoma of the head of pancreas
   D. Sclerosing cholangitis

106. **Cigarette smoking may predispose to all** *except*
   A. Hepatocellular carcinoma   B. Periampullary carcinoma
   C. Cholangiocarcinoma   D. Carcinoma of pancreas

107. **Which is not an extrahepatic manifestation of hepatitis B virus infection**
   A. Polymyalgia rheumatica
   B. Essential mixed cryoglobulinaemia
   C. Guillain-Barré syndrome
   D. Fibrosing alveolitis

108. **Which one is false in granulomatous hepatitis**
   A. Mild, firm hepatomegaly
   B. Jaundice
   C. Sarcoidosis may be an aetiology
   D. Liver biopsy is diagnostic

109. **All are metabolic causes of cirrhosis of liver** *except*
   A. Type IV glycogenesis   B. Galactosaemia
   C. Homocystinurias   D. Wilson's disease

110. **Acutely tender liver is found in all** *except*
   A. Congestive cardiac failure   B. Amoebic liver abscess
   C. Carcinoma of liver   D. Haemangioma of liver

111. **Amoebic typhlitis is the inflammation of**
   A. Hepatic capsule leading to perihepatitis
   B. Hepatic flexure of large intestine
   C. Sigmoido-rectal junction
   D. Caecum

112. **Secondary carcinoma of liver should not have**
   A. Malignant ascites   B. Splenomegaly
   C. Jaundice   D. Knobbly liver

113. **Commonest cause of portal hypertension is**
   A. Acute viral hepatitis   B. Chronic active hepatitis
   C. Cirrhosis of liver   D. Carcinoma of liver

Ans: 105-A 106-C 107-D 108-B 109-C 110-D 111-D 112-B 113-C

114. Treatment modalities of Wilson's disease include all *except*
    A. Tetrathiomolybdate
    B. Penicillamine
    C. Colchicine
    D. Elemental zinc

115. Most consistent clinical finding in haemochromatosis is
    A. Increased skin pigmentation
    B. Hepatomegaly
    C. Arthropathy
    D. Hypogonadism

116. Rapid diminution in the size of liver is seen in
    A. Cholangiohepatitis
    B. Fulminant hepatic failure
    C. Carcinoma of liver
    D. Acute alcoholic hepatitis

117. The Kayser-Fleischer ring is
    A. Broader laterally and medially
    B. The inferior pole of cornea is first affected
    C. Copper deposition in Descemet's membrane
    D. Hampers vision

118. Definitive test for diagnosis of haemochromatosis is
    A. Plasma iron >300 µg/dl
    B. Liver biopsy
    C. TIBC < 200 µg/dl
    D. Hepatic iron index >1.5

119. Superficial venous flow in portal hypertension is
    A. Away from the umbilicus
    B. Below upwards
    C. Towards umbilicus
    D. Above downwards

120. Which of the following is false regarding haemochromatosis
    A. Pancreatic iron deposition leads to diabetes
    B. Most common cardiac manifestation is congestive heart failure
    C. Melanin and iron deposition gives rise to bronzing of skin
    D. Hypogonadism results from iron deposition in testes

121. Commonest cause of post-transfusion hepatitis is
    A. Hepatitis B
    B. Hepatitis C
    C. Hepatitis D
    D. Hepatitis E

122. Kayser-Fleischer like ring is found in all *except*
    A. Cryptogenic cirrhosis
    B. Chronic active hepatitis
    C. Prolonged cholestasis
    D. Chronic biliary cirrhosis

123. Commonest hepatic lesion in haemochromatosis is
    A. Fatty liver
    B. Macronodular cirrhosis
    C. Micronodular cirrhosis
    D. Haemosiderosis

Ans: 114-C 115-B 116-B 117-C 118-B 119-A 120-D 121-B 122-B 123-B

124. All are characteristic features of Wilson's disease *except*
    A. Chorea
    B. Sensory loss
    C. Grimacing
    D. Slurred speech

125. Streptokinase is nowadays tried in the treatment of
    A. Sclerosing cholangitis
    B. Haemangioma of liver
    C. Matastasis in liver
    D. Budd-Chiari syndrome

126. Corticosteroid may be given in
    A. Alcoholic hepatitis
    B. Acute viral hepatitis B
    C. Rifampicin-induced hepatitis
    D. Copper sulphate poisoning

127. Absolute contraindication for liver biopsy is
    A. Cirrhosis of liver
    B. Cholestasis
    C. Haemangioma of liver
    D. Amoebic liver abscess

128. Which one of the following is false regarding primary biliary cirrhosis
    A. Female preponderance
    B. Starts with pruritus
    C. Moderate to severe jaundice
    D. Clubbing

129. Most common cause of fulminant hepatic failure is
    A. Chronic active hepatitis
    B. Alcoholic hepatitis
    C. Drug-induced hepatitis
    D. Acute viral hepatitis

130. All of the following may develop into chronic active hepatitis *except*
    A. Methyldopa
    B. Captopril
    C. Isoniazid
    D. Oxyphenisatin

131. Which one of the following is true regarding pre-sinusoidal portal hypertension
    A. Blocked hepatic vein
    B. Raised wedged hepatic venous pressure
    C. Congenital hepatic fibrosis is an example
    D. Commonest cause of portal hypertension

132. Congestive gastropathy in portal hypertension is best treated by
    A. Terlipressin
    B. Somatostatin
    C. Propranolol
    D. Nitroglycerines

Ans: 124-B 125-D 126-A 127-C 128-C 129-D 130-B 131-C 132-C

133. **Which of the following is not true in lupoid hepatitis**
    A. Cushingoid face
    B. Associated with other autoimmune diseases
    C. High risk of developing into hepatoma
    D. ANF is positive in majority

134. **Which of the following is false regarding Gaucher's disease**
    A. Pre-malignant
    B. Hepatosplenomegaly
    C. High serum acid phosphatase level
    D. Elevated serum angiotensin-converting enzyme

135. **Which indicates chronicity in hepatitis B virus infection**
    A. HBeAg   B. Anti-HBs
    C. DNA polymerase   D. IgG anti-HBc

136. **Commonest cause of jaundice in pregnancy is**
    A. Toxaemia of pregnancy
    B. Acute fatty liver of pregnancy
    C. Acute viral hepatitis
    D. Use of hepatotoxic drugs

137. **Acute viral hepatitis may develop from all of the following** *except*
    A. Yellow fever   B. Herpes zoster virus
    C. Infectious mononucleosis D. Cytomegalovirus

138. **Commonest cause of hepatoma is**
    A. α_1-antitrypsin deficiency   B. Haemochromatosis
    C. Alcohol   D. Cirrhosis of liver

139. **Tumour of liver found predominantly in females is**
    A. Adenoma   B. Hepatocellular carcinoma
    C. Angiosarcoma   D. Hepatoblastoma

140. **All of the following are prognostic factors in acute pancreatitis** *except*
    A. Hyperamylasia   B. Hypoalbuminaemia
    C. Hyperglycaemia   D. Hypocalcaemia

141. **Commonest organism causing pyogenic liver abscess is**
    A. Anaerobes   B. Staphylococci
    C. *Streptococcus faecalis* D. *E. coli*

Ans: 133-C 134-A 135-D 136-C 137-B 138-D 139-A 140-A 141-D

142. **Mallory hyaline is absent in**
    A. Amoebic hepatitis
    B. Alcoholic hepatitis
    C. Amiodarone-induced hepatitis
    D. Indian childhood cirrhosis

143. **Which of the following is false in Caroli's disease**
    A. Segmental dilatation of intrahepatic bile ducts
    B. Familial
    C. Congenital hepatic fibrosis may be associated with
    D. Cholangiocarcinoma may be a complication

144. **Most common benign tumour of liver is**
    A. Focal nodular hyperplasia
    B. Adenomas
    C. Haemangiomas
    D. Nodular regenerative hyperplasia

145. **Weil's disease is associated with**
    A. Jaundice in all
    B. Severe muscle pain
    C. Absence of renal involvement
    D. Leucopenia with lymphocytosis

146. **Calcification of spleen is seen in**
    A. Tropical splenomegaly syndrome
    B. Thalassaemia
    C. Malarial spleen
    D. Hydatid cyst

147. **In HBV infection, which serological maker is present in the 'window period' as an evidence of recent HBV infection**
    A. Hb_eAg B. IgG anti-HBc
    C. IgM anti-HBc   D. HBV DNA

148. **Regarding non-alcoholic steatohepatosis (NASH), all are true** *except*
    A. Occasionally progresses to cirrhosis and liver failure
    B. Typically occurs in overweight, diabetic, hyperlipidaemic subjects
    C. Jejunoileal bypass may be an aetiology
    D. Glucocorticoid helps cure

149. **Acute pancreatitis is caused by all** *except*
    A. Hypertriglyceridaemia   B. ACE inhibitors
    C. Hypocalcaemia   D. Blunt trauma

Ans: 142-A 143-B 144-C 145-B 146-D 147-C 148-D 149-C

150. **Commonest type of hepatitis epidemic in India is**
    A. Hepatitis A
    B. Hepatitis B
    C. Hepatitis C
    D. Hepatitis E

151. **In acute infection with HBV, first thing to appear or rise in blood is**
    A. HbsAg
    B. Anti-HBs
    C. SGPT
    D. Bilirubin

152. **Which of the following reflects the best prognostic parameter of hepatocellular function**
    A. SGPT
    B. Alkaline phosphatase
    C. Serum bilirubin
    D. Prothrombin time

153. **The presenting feature of non-cirrhotic portal fibrosis is**
    A. Upper GI bleeding
    B. Ascites
    C. Hepatocellular failure
    D. Hepatomegaly

154. **Continued infectivity in HBV infection is diagnosed by**
    A. IgM anti-HBc
    B. HBsAg
    C. HBV DNA
    D. Anti-HBs

155. **Most common cause of Budd-Chiari syndrome is**
    A. Paroxysmal nocturnal haemoglobinuria
    B. Oral contraceptives
    C. Valve in hepatic veins
    D. Hepatoma

156. **All are associated with raised serum amylase** *except*
    A. Diabetic ketoacidosis
    B. Ruptured ectopic pregnancy
    C. Bleeding peptic ulcer
    D. Peritonitis

157. **Which vitamin deficiency occurs in obstructive jaundice**
    A. Folic acid
    B. Vitamin A
    C. Vitamin C
    D. Vitamin B_{12}

158. **Which of the following is false regarding acrodermatitis entero-pathica**
    A. Desquamating skin lesion
    B. Severe diarrhoea
    C. Zinc deficiency
    D. Associated with thymic hyperplasia

Ans: 150-D 151-A 152-D 153-A 154-C 155-C 156-C 157-B 158-D

159. **In acute HBV infection, spherical Dane particle has the size of**

    A. 22 nm
    B. 27 nm
    C. 42 nm
    D. 48 nm

160. **↑ α_1-fetoprotein is found in all *except***

    A. Oesophageal atresia
    B. Postmaturity
    C. Spina bifida
    D. Hepatocellular carcinoma

161. **Presence of caput medusae denies the diagnosis of**

    A. Non-cirrhotic portal fibrosis
    B. Budd-Chiari syndrome
    C. Extrahepatic portal vein thrombosis
    D. Laennec's cirrhosis

162. **Morphine is virtually contraindicated in**

    A. Acute myocardial infarction
    B. Terminal cancer pain
    C. Biliary colic
    D. Acute left ventricular failure

163. **Example of calcivirus is**

    A. Hepatitis A virus
    B. Hepatitis B virus
    C. Hepatitis C virus
    D. Hepatitis E virus

164. **Medical dissolution of gallstones is done by all *except***

    A. Methyl tertiary butyl ether
    B. Lithocholic acid
    C. Monooctanoin
    D. Ursodeoxycholic acid

165. **Non-alcoholic steatohepatosis (NASH) may be produced by all *except***

    A. Massive dose of oestrogen
    B. Amiodarone
    C. Nifedipine
    D. Tetracycline

166. **Hepatopulmonary syndrome is manifested by all *except***

    A. Cyanosis
    B. Widespread intrapulmonary vascular dilatations
    C. Orthopnoea
    D. Increased alveolar-arterial oxygen gradient

167. **Minimal hepatic encephalopathy is classically diagnosed by**

    A. Psychometric study
    B. EEC
    C. Evoked potential study
    D. MRI of brain

Ans: 159-C 160-B 161-C 162-C 163-D 164-B 165-D 166-C 167-A

168. **Mid-zonal necrosis of liver is caused by**
    A. Phosphorus poisoning
    B. Eclampsia
    C. Yellow fever
    D. Carbon tetrachloride

169. **Predominant unconjugated bilirubin is seen in all *except***
    A. Breakdown of myoglobin
    B. Rotor syndrome
    C. Ineffective erythropoiesis
    D. Breakdown of haemoglobin

170. **Pancreatic exocrine insufficiency happens to begin, when**
    A. 40% of pancreas is lost
    B. 60% of pancreas is lost
    C. 75% of pancreas is lost
    D. 90% of pancreas is lost

171. **Pregnancy predisposes to all *except***
    A. Acute hepatic failure
    B. Chronic hepatitis
    C. Steatosis
    D. Cholestasis

172. **Portal hypertension associated with soft liver suggests**
    A. Budd-Chiari syndrome
    B. Extrahepatic obstruction
    C. Non-cirrhotic portal fibrosis
    D. Cirrhosis of liver

173. **Splenic dullness can be percussed by all *except***
    A. Castell's method
    B. Nixon's method
    C. Osler's method
    D. Barkun's method of Traube's space percussion

174. **'Sago spleen' is found in**
    A. Chronic myeloid leukaemia
    B. Felty's syndrome
    C. Chronic active hepatitis
    D. Focal amyloidosis

175. **Fatty liver is not characteristic of**
    A. Indian childhood cirrhosis
    B. Reye's syndrome
    C. Protein-calorie malnutrition
    D. Total parenteral nutrition

176. **Which is not an indication of liver transplantation**
    A. Hereditary oxalosis
    B. Tyrosinaemia
    C. Haemangioma of liver
    D. Primary sclerosing cholangitis

177. **Which is the most sensitive test to diagnose hepatopulmonary syndrome**
    A. CT scan of liver
    B. Contrast-enhanced echocardiography
    C. MRI scan of liver
    D. Pulmonary angiography

Ans: 168-C 169-B 170-D 171-B 172-B 173-C 174-D 175-A 176-C 177-B

178. **Lardaceous spleen is seen in**

    A. Chronic myeloid leukaemia
    B. Chronic kala-azar
    C. Subacute bacterial endocarditis
    D. Diffuse amyloidosis

179. **Autoimmune pancreatitis is synonymous with all** *except*

    A. Non-alcoholic destructive pancreatitis
    B. Tumefactive pancreatitis
    C. Hereditary pancreatitis
    D. Sclerosing pancreatitis

180. **All are 'medical causes of acute abdomen'** *except*

    A. Apical pneumonia
    B. Sickle cell anaemia
    C. Acute myocardial infarction
    D. Lead poisoning

181. **Hepatic granuloma may develop from**

    A. Allopurinol   B. Risperidone
    C. Valproic acid   D. Oxyphenisatin

182. **Which of the following is false regarding autoimmune hepatitis**

    A. Hyperglobulinaemia is common
    B. AST and ALT levels fluctuate within 100–1000 units
    C. Very high bilirubin level
    D. Hypoalbuminaemia is very active disease

183. **Which of the following is not an 'absolute' contraindication in hepatic transplantation**

    A. Untreated sepsis   B. AIDS
    C. Renal failure   D. Active alcohol abuse

184. **Sclerosing cholangitis may be associated with all** *except*

    A. Pseudotumour of the orbit
    B. Fibrosis of the lung
    C. Autoimmune pancreatitis
    D. Riedel's struma

Ans: 178-D 179-C 180-A 181-A 182-C 183-C 184-B

Cardiology

1. **Pericardial rub is best audible in all** *except*

   A. By pressing the chest piece of stethoscope
   B. After holding the breath
   C. On the left side of lower sternum
   D. In lying down position

2. **Slow rising pulse is a feature of**

   A. Endotoxic shock
   B. AS
   C. MS
   D. Constrictive pericarditis

3. **Pulsus alternans is produced by**

   A. Pericardial effusion
   B. Left-sided heart failure
   C. Chronic obstructive airway disease
   D. Pulmonary thromboembolism

4. **Central cyanosis is not found in**

   A. Acute pulmonary oedema
   B. Fallot's tetralogy
   C. Left-to-right shunt
   D. Transposition of great vessels

5. **Which of the following is not a cause of sinus bradycardia**

   A. Myxoedema
   B. Complete heart block
   C. Hypothermia
   D. Obstructive jaundice

6. **Regrading neck venous pulsation, which is false**

   A. Undulating
   B. Better felt than seen
   C. Becomes prominent on lying down
   D. There are two negative waves

7. **Unilateral clubbing is found in all** *except*

   A. Presubclavian coarctation of aorta
   B. Aneurysm of subclavian artery
   C. Arteriovenous fistula of brachial vessels
   D. Takayasu's disease

Ans: 1-D 2-B 3-B 4-C 5-B 6-B 7-D

8. Water-hammer pulse is present, when pulse pressure is at least above
   A. 30 mm Hg
   B. 80 mm Hg
   C. 40 mm Hg
   D. 60 mm Hg

9. All are cardiovascular features of severe anaemia *except*
   A. Water-hammer pulse
   B. Tapping apex
   C. Cardiomegaly
   D. Systolic murmur over the pulmonary area

10. Radiofemoral delay is a feature of all *except*
    A. Aortoarteritis
    B. Coarctation of aorta
    C. Unfolding of aorta
    D. Atherosclerosis of aorta

11. Giant a-wave in neck vein is seen in
    A. Left atrial myxoma
    B. Constrictive pericarditis
    C. Pulmonary hypertension
    D. Atrial fibrillation

12. Clubbing is not a feature of
    A. Fallot's tetralogy
    B. Left atrial myxoma
    C. Right-to-left shunt
    D. Acute bacterial endocarditis

13. Left parasternal heave is diagnostic of
    A. Left ventricular hypertrophy
    B. Right atrial hypertrophy
    C. Right ventricular hypertrophy
    D. Hypertrophic cardiomyopathy

14. Pulsus bisferiens is found in
    A. Combined AS and AI
    B. Combined MS and AS
    C. Combined AI and MI
    D. Combined MS and MI

15. v-wave in JVP becomes prominent in
    A. Tricuspid incompetence
    B. Cardiac tamponade
    C. Ventricular tachycardia
    D. Right atrial myxoma

16. Which of the following is false regarding oedema in congestive cardiac failure
    A. Initially noticed in the morning
    B. Starts in the dependent par'
    C. Pitting oedema
    D. Sacral oedema in non-ambulatory patients

Ans: 8-D 9-B 10-C 11-C 12-D 13-C 14-A 15-A 16-A

17. **Which does not produce regularly irregular pulse**
    A. 2nd degree heart block
    B. Atrial fibrillation
    C. Extrasystoles
    D. Sinus arrhythmia

18. **Sudden death may occur in**
    A. AS
    B. ASD
    C. Constrictive pericarditis
    D. PDA

19. **Digitalis toxicity is associated with all *except***
    A. Wenckebach block
    B. Ventricular bigeminy
    C. Paroxysmal atrial tachycardia with block
    D. Mobitz type II block

20. **The sound best audible by bell of stethoscope is**
    A. S_2
    B. Venous hum
    C. Ejection click
    D. Opening snap

21. **Long tubular heart in X-ray chest is found in all *except***
    A. Isolated levocardia
    B. Addison's disease
    C. Emphysema
    D. Sheehan's syndrome

22. **Electrical alternans in EGG is seen in**
    A. Pericardial effusion
    B. Left ventricular failure
    C. Digitalis toxicity
    D. Wenckebach block

23. **Ideally, the connecting tube of stethoscope should be**
    A. 8 inch long
    B. 12 inch long
    C. 18 inch long
    D. 22 inch long

24. **RBBB with left axis deviation in ECG is characteristically seen in**
    A. VSD
    B. Ostium primum ASD
    C. PDA
    D. Fallot's tetralogy

25. **Sphygmomanometer cannot diagnose**
    A. Pulsus paradoxus
    B. Pulsus alternans
    C. Water-hammer pulse
    D. Pulsus bigeminus

26. **Short PR interval in ECG is characteristic of**
    A. Rheumatic carditis
    B. Digitalis toxicity
    C. W-P-W syndrome
    D. Ischaemic heart disease (IHD)

Ans: 17-B 18-A 19-D 20-B 21-A 22-A 23-B 24-B 25-D 26-C

27. **Stethoscope was invented by**
    A. Laennec   B. Osler
    C. Babinski   D. Korotkoff

28. **U-wave in EGG is characteristically found in**
    A. Hyperkalaemia   B. Hyponatraemia
    C. Hypocalcaemia   D. Hypokalaemia

29. **All of the following produce systemic hypertension *except***
    A. Polycystic kidney disease
    B. Phaeochromocytoma
    C. Addison's disease
    D. Conn's syndrome

30. **Classical JVP finding in cardiac tamponade is**
    A. Prominent a-wave   B. Prominent x-descent
    C. Prominent y-descent   D. Small v-wave

31. **Left atrial failure is featured by all *except***
    A. Dependent oedema
    B. Paroxysmal nocturnal dyspnoea
    C. Fine crepitations at lung bases
    D. Gallop rhythm

32. **All are bedside differential diagnosis of MS *except***
    A. Carey Coombs murmur   B. Left atrial myxoma
    C. Austin Flint murmur   D. Mitral valve prolapse syndrome

33. **The least common complication of MS is**
    A. Cerebral thrombosis   B. Subacute bacterial endocarditis
    C. Pulmonary hypertension   D. Atrial fibrillation

34. **Chinically, severity of MS is best assessed by**
    A. Diastolic shock
    B. Proximity of S_2-opening snap gap
    C. Paroxysmal nocturnal dyspnoea (PND)
    D. Shorter duration of mid-diastolic murmur

35. **Opening snap is**
    A. Low-pitched
    B. Best heard with the bell of stethoscope
    C. Best heard in standing position
    D. Present in late diastole

Ans: 27-A 28-D 29-C 30-B 31-A 32-D 33-B 34-B 35-C

36. Haemoptysis may be found in
- A. Left ventricular failure
- B. Right ventricular failure
- C. Pulmonary stenosis
- D. Left-to-right shurt

37. All are features of acute attack of PND *except*
- A. Peripheral cyanosis
- B. Raised JVP
- C. Ashen-grey pallor
- D. S_3 gallop rhythm

38. Which chamber of heart fails first in MS
- A. Right atrium
- B. Right ventricle
- C. Left atrium
- D. Left ventricle

39. Which is false regarding juvenile mitral stenosis
- A. Pin-point mitral valve
- B. Occurs below 18 years
- C. Atrial fibrillation is commonly seen
- D. Mitral valve calcification is uncommon

40. In critical MS, the mitral valve orifice is
- A. $< 6 \ cm^2$
- B. $< 4 \ cm^2$
- C. $< 2 \ cm^2$
- D. $< 1 \ cm^2$

41. Maral flush is found in all *except*
- A. Mitral stenosis
- B. Myxoedema
- C. Carcinoid syndrome
- D. Systemic lupus erythematosus

42. All of the following are causes of intermittent claudication *except*
- A. Leriche's syndrome
- B. Lumbar canal stenosis
- C. Peripheral neuropathy
- D. Buerger's disease

43. Indications for closed mitral valvotomy include all *except*
- A. Absence of valvular calcification
- B. Absence of left atrial thrombus
- C. Pure mitral stenosis
- D. Restenosis cases

44. Roth spot is found in all *except*
- A. Aplastic anaemia
- B. Acute leukaemia
- C. Takayasu's disease
- D. Subacute bacterial endocarditis

45. Hill's sign is diagnostic of
- A. AI
- B. MS
- C. AS
- D. MI

Ans: 36-A 37-A 38-C 39-C 40-D 41-D 42-C 43-D 44-C 45-A

46. **Which of the following gives rise to heaving apex beat**
    A. MS   B. MI
    C. AS   D. AI

47. **Concentric left ventricular hypertrophy (LVH) is usually found in**
    A. Ischaemic heart disease   B. Cardiomyopathy
    C. Coarctation of aorta   D. Severe anaemia

48. **Mental retardation, squint, idiopathic hypercalcaemia may be associated with "stenosis' of**
    A. Pulmonary valve   B. Mitral valve
    C. Aortic valve   D. Tricuspid valve

49. **Which of the following does not produce continuous murmur**
    A. Peripheral pulmonary stenosis
    B. Ruptured sinus of Valsalva
    C. Aortopulmonary window
    D. Pulmonary arteriovenous fistula

50. **Elfin facies (pointed chin; cupid's bow-like upper lip, upturned nose) may be seen in**
    A. Supravalvular AS   B. Lutembacher syndrome
    C. Ebstein's anomaly   D. Infundibular PS

51. **Which of the following does not lead to Eisenmenger's syndrome**
    A. Coarctation of aorta   B. PDA
    C. ASD   D. VSD

52. **Seagull murmur is not a feature of**
    A. Acute myocardial infarction
    B. Acute rheumatic fever
    C. Subacute bacterial endocarditis
    D. Floppy mitral valve

53. **AI with low pulse pressure is found in all *except***
    A. AI with tight PS
    B. AI with systemic hypertension
    C. AI with CCF
    D. Acutely developing AI

54. **Which of the following is not an aetiology of MI**
    A. Pseudoxanthoma elasticum   B. Osteoarthritis
    C. Osteogenesis imperfecta   D. Ehlers-Danlos syndrome

Ans: 46-C 47-C 48-C 49-A 50-A 51-A 52-D 53-A 54-B

55. **Bedside diagnosis of a classical case of SBE does not include**

    A   Cafe-au-lait pallor
    B. Macroscopic haematuria
    C. Clubbing
    D. Splenomegaly

56. **Which one is false regarding floppy mitral valve**

    A. Most of the patients are asymptomatic
    B. High-pitched late systolic murmur
    C. More common in females
    D. Early systolic click

57. **Which of the following does not produce 'fleeting' arthritis**

    A. SLE   B. Rheumatic arthritis
    C. Felty's syndrome   D. Viral arthritis

58. **Murmur of floppy mitral valve increases with all *except***

    A. Valsalva manoeuvre   B. Squatting
    C. Amyl nitrite inhalation   D. Standing

59. **Commonest organism producing acute bacterial endocarditis is**

    A. *Streptococcus viridans*   B. *Staphylococcus aureus*
    C. *Streptococcus faecalis*   D. *Pneumococcus*

60. **Cardiac percussion is important in**

    A. Acute myocardial infarction B. Emphysema
    C. Myocarditis   D. Cardiomyopathy

61. **Which of the following is not included in 'minor manifestation' of Jones criteria in rheumatic fever**

    A. Prolonged PR interval   B. Arthralgia
    C. Increased ESR   D. Elevated ASO titre

62. **The ESR may be very low in all *except***

    A. Congestive cardiac failure
    B. Sickle cell anaemia
    C. Pregnancy
    D. Polycythaemia

63. **Which is of the following not a 'major manifestation' of Jones criteria in rheumatic fever**

    A. Chorea   B. Erythema nodosum
    C. Subcutaneous nodule   D. Polyarthritis

Ans: 55-B 56-D 57-C 58-B 59-B 60-B 61-D 62-C 63-B

64. The ESR may be 'zero' in

A. Old age
B. Vasculitis
C. Afibrinogenaemia
D. SLE

65. Which of the following is not recognised to be an acute phase reactant

A. Alpha fetoprotein
B. Orosomucoid
C. Caeruloplasmin
D. Haptoglobulin

66. All are examples of congenital cyanotic heart disease *except*

A. Ebstein's anomaly
B. Anomalous origin of coronary artery
C. Fallot's tetralogy
D. Single ventricle

67. Lutembacher's syndrome is

A. ASD plus AI
B. VSD plus MS
C. ASD plus MI
D. ASD plus MS

68. Differential diagnoses of ASD at the bedside are all *except*

A. Total anomalous pulmonary venous connection (TAPVC)
B. Idiopathic pulmonary artery dilatation
C. PDA
D. Pulmonary stenosis

69. 'Fallot's pentalogy' is Fallot's tetralogy plus

A. ASD
B. PDA
C. Associated LVH
D. AS

70. All are commonly associated with ASD *except*

A. Ellis-van Creveld syndrome
B. Holt-Oram syndrome
C. Down's syndrome
D. Trisomy 18

71. Coarctation of aorta may be associated with all *except*

A. Polycystic kidney
B. Berry aneurysm
C. Bicuspid aortic valve
D. Aortic arch syndrome

72. Commonest congenital heart disease is

A. ASD
B. VSD
C. Bicuspid aortic valve
D. Fallot's tetralogy

Ans: 64-C 65-A 66-B 67-D 68-C 69-A 70-D 71-D 72-C

73. **All are true in severe PS** *except*

    A. The ejection click goes away from S_1
    B. Intensity of murmur is maximum towards S_2
    C. Gap between A_2 and P_2 is increased
    D. A_2 is gradually rounded by the murmur

74. **Aortic arch syndrome is not associated with**

    A. Diminished pulses in upper extremity
    B. Disturbances in vision
    C. Intermittent claudication
    D. Systemic hypertension

75. **Which of the following drugs is not used in hypoxic spells of Fallot's tetralogy**

    A. Phenylephrine
    B. Amiodarone
    C. Propranolol
    D. Morphine

76. **The disease with male preponderance is**

    A. Coarctation of aorta
    B. Primary pulmonary hypertension
    C. SLE
    D. PDA

77. **The '3-sign' in chest roentgenogram diagnoses**

    A. PS
    B. VSD
    C. Coarctation of aorta
    D. AS

78. **Varying intensity of S_1 is found in all** *except*

    A. Nodal rhythm
    B. Ventricular tachycardia
    C. Complete heart block
    D. Atrial fibrillation

79. **Double apex in hypertrophic cardiomyopathy is mainly due to**

    A. Palpable S_4
    B. Muscle tremor
    C. Palpable opening snap
    D. Palpable S_3

80. **Muffled S_1 is found in all** *except*

    A. Digitalis overdose
    B. Tachycardia
    C. Mitral valve calcification
    D. Left atrial failure

81. **'Diastolic shock' is not found in**

    A. Chronic cor pulmonale
    B. PS
    C. MS
    D. VSD

Ans: 73-A 74-C 75-B 76-A 77-C 78-A 79-A 80-B 81-B

82. **Loud A_2 is present in**
    A. Pulmonary hypertension
    B. Calcified aortic valve
    C. Aortitis
    D. Unfolding of aorta

83. **Atrial myxomas may be associated with all *except***
    A. Pyrexia
    B. Splenomegaly
    C. Clubbing
    D. High ESR

84. **Which is not a cause of wide and fixed splitting of S_2**
    A. Massive pulmonary thromboembolism
    B. Right ventricular pacing
    C. ASD
    D. Left ventricular failure

85. **Endomyocardial fibrosis may be due to**
    A. Tapioca
    B. Coffee
    C. Bush tea
    D. Aflatoxin

86. **S_4 is not associated with**
    A. Aortic stenosis
    B. Hypertrophic cardiomyopathy
    C. Chronic mitral regurgitation
    D. Systemic hypertension

87. **Intracardiac calcification usually indicates**
    A. Chronic constrictive pericarditis
    B. Subacute bacterial endocarditis
    C. Rheumatic valve
    D. Mural thrombus

88. **S_3 or S_4 is best auscultated**
    A. With the diaphragm of stethoscope
    B. In standing position
    C. Stethoscope placed lightly over the apex
    D. Anywhere in the precordium

89. **Incidence of infective endocarditis is least in**
    A. MI
    B. PDA
    C. ASD
    D. VSD

90. **Pulsus paradoxus is seen in all *except***
    A. Acute severe asthma
    B. Cardiac tamponade
    C. Constrictive pericarditis
    D. Dilated cardiomyopathy

Ans: 82-C 83-B 84-D 85-A 86-C 87-C 88-C 89-C 90-D

91. Sudden death may occur in all of the following *except*
    A. Atrial fibrillation
    B. Massive myocardial infarction
    C. Ventricular fibrillation
    D. Massive pulmonary thromboembolism

92. S_3 may be present in all *except*
    A. Hypertrophic cardiomyopathy
    B. Pregnancy
    C. Hyperkinetic circulatory states
    D. Athletes

93. Myocarditis may be found in all *except*
    A. HIV infection   B. Toxoplasma infection
    C. Diphtheria   D. Ascariasis

94. Echocardiography can diagnose the presence of pericardial fluid as little as
    A. 5 ml   B. 15 ml
    C. 25 ml   D. 100 ml

95. All are helpful in the treatment of hypertrophic cardiomyopathy *except*
    A. ACE-inhibitors
    B. Amiodarone
    C. Surgical myotomy of the septum
    D. Propranolol

96. The S_2 in Fallot's tetralogy
    A. Shows narrow split   B. Having wide split
    C. Remains single   D. Shows reverse split

97. Cardiomyopathy may follow treatment with
    A. Chloramphenicol   B. Doxorubicin
    C. Methotrexate   D. Allopurinol

98. Normal blood volume in an adult male is approximately
    A. 50 ml/kg of body weight   B. 60 ml/kg of body weight
    C. 70 ml/kg of body weight   D. 85 ml/kg of body weight

99. Carey Coombs murmur is found in
    A. Pulmonary hypertension   B. AI
    C. Acute rheumatic fever   D. MS

Ans: 91-A 92-A 93-D 94-B 95-A 96-C 97-B 98-C 99-C

100. **Which of the following is not advocated in the treatment of acute pulmonary oedema**
   A. Diuretics
   B. Trendelenburg position
   C. Morphine
   D. Rotating tourniquets

101. **Kussmaul's sign is present in**
   A. Hypertrophic cardiomyopathy
   B. Right ventricular infarction
   C. Myocarditis
   D. Pregnancy

102. **All are class I antiarrhythmic drugs** *except*
   A. Disopyramide
   B. Flecainide
   C. Verapamil
   D. Quinidine

103. **Cardiac involvement is absent in**
   A. Facio-scapulo-humeral dystrophy
   B. Myotonic dystrophy
   C. Duchenne type muscular dystrophy
   D. Friedreich's ataxia

104. **All of the following may have unidigital clubbing** *except*
   A. Tophaceous gout
   B. Trauma
   C. Sarcoidosis
   D. Cervical rib

105. **Digitalis toxicity is precipitated by all** *except*
   A. Old age
   B. Hypokalaemia
   C. Renal failure
   D. Hepatic encephalopathy

106. **Cannon wave in the neck vein is seen in**
   A. Complete heart block
   B. Constrictive pericarditis
   C. Tricuspid incompetence
   D. Right atrial myxoma

107. **Left ventricular hypertrophy is not associated with**
   A. AS
   B. AI
   C. MS
   D. MI

108. **Which of the following is not found in constrictive pericarditis**
   A. Pulmonary oedema
   B. Raised JVP
   C. Ascites
   D. Pulsus paradoxus

109. **Prolonged QT interval in EGG is found in all** *except*
   A. Quinidine therapy
   B. Hypothermia
   C. Vagal stimulation
   D. Hypocalcaemia

Ans: 100-B 101-B 102-C 103-A 104-D 105-D 106-A 107-C 108-A 109-C

110. **During cardiopulmonary resuscitation, external defibrillation by DC shock is done with**
    A. 50 Joules
    B. 100 Joules
    C. 200 Joules
    D. 400 Joules

111. **Differential cyanosis is found in**
    A. Fallot's tetralogy
    B. Transposition of great vessels
    C. VSD
    D. Ebstein's anomaly

112. **Very close differential diagnosis of constrictive pericarditis at the bedside is**
    A. Congestive cardiac failure
    B. Superior mediastinal syndrome
    C. Left ventricular failure
    D. Cirrhosis of liver

113. **All are features of pericardial tamponade *except***
    A. Orthopnoea
    B. Pulsatile liver
    C. Hypotension
    D. Raised JVP

114. **Acute myocardial infarction of posterior wall of left ventricle will show in the ECG**
    A. Deep Q waves in V_{1-6}
    B. ST depression and tall R wave in V_{1-4}
    C. ST elevation in II, III, aVF
    D. ST elevation in I, aVL, V_6

115. **Which one of the following is false regarding Austin Flint murmur**
    A. Found in severe AI
    B. Having loud S_1
    C. Mid-diastolic murmur
    D. Absence of thrill

116. **Acute subendocardial infarction will have ECG finding**
    A. Prominent ST elevation
    B. Deep Q wave
    C. Deep symmetrical T wave inversion
    D. Height of R wave maximum in V_6

117. **'Auscultatory gap' in BP measurement is**
    A. Present in all hypertensives
    B. Should be ignored
    C. Related to diastolic BP
    D. As a result of venous distension

118. **All of the following are common arrhythmias developing from AMI *except***
    A. Sinus arrhythmia
    B. Ventricular tachycardia
    C. Wenckebach heart block
    D. Accelerated idioventricular rhythm

Ans: 110-C 111-B 112-D 113-B 114-B 115-B 116-C 117-D 118-A

119. **Paroxysmal hypertension is classically found in**
    A. Coarctation of aorta
    B. Eclampsia
    C. Renal artery stenosis
    D. Phaeochromocytoma

120. **Regarding Kerley's B lines, all of the following are true** *except*
    A. Found in basal region
    B. May be seen in pre-oedema stage
    C. Its presence indicates left atrial pressure >10 mm Hg
    D. MS is a recognised cause

121. **Cardiac arrest may be due to**
    A. Multiple ectopics
    B. Atrial flutter
    C. Pulseless ventricular tachycardia
    D. Wenckebach block

122. **A pericardial friction rub may have any of the components** *except*
    A. Presystolic
    B. Mid-diastolic
    C. Early diastolic
    D. Systolic

123. **Torsade de pointes is associated with**
    A. Increased QT interval
    B. Increased duration of QRS complex
    C. Presence of J-wave
    D. Increased PR interval

124. **The murmur of MS is**
    A. Increased by amyl nitrite inhalation
    B. High-pitched
    C. Early diastolic
    D. With radiation towards left axilla

125. **Which one of the following is a centrally-acting antihypertensive drug**
    A. Prazosin
    B. Methyldopa
    C. Amiloride
    D. Hydralazine

126. **Diagnosis of AMI within 6 hrs depends on**
    A. CPK MB_2/CPK $MB_1 \geq 1.5$
    B. Increased LDH_3
    C. Rise of SGPT > 250 IU/L
    D. Inverted T wave in ECG

Ans: 119-D 120-C 121-C 122-B 123-A 124-A 125-B 126-A

127. **Which one of the following is false regarding atrial fibrillation**
    A. 'f' waves in neck vein
    B. Atrial rate is 350–400/min
    C. Ventricular rate is 100–150/min
    D. Pulse deficit is >10

128 **The Keith-Wagener-Barker classification for retinal changes is meant for**
    A. Diabetes mellitus
    B. Aortoarteritis
    C. Systemic hypertension
    D. Takayasu's disease

129. **S_1 S_2 S_3 syndrome in ECG is seen in**
    A. Hypothermia
    B. Left ventricular hypertrophy
    C. Digitalis toxicity
    D. Chronic cor pulmonale

130. **Retrosternal chest pain classically occurs in all *except***
    A. Acute mediastinitis
    B. Dissecting aneurysm
    C. Bornholm disease
    D. Unstable angina

131. **Delta wave in ECG is found in**
    A. Sick sinus syndrome
    B. Hypothermia
    C. W-P-W syndrome
    D. Hyperkalaemia

132. **CPK-MB is increased in all *except***
    A. Myocarditis
    B. Rhabdomyolysis
    C. Post-AMI
    D. Post-electrical cardioversion

133. **Which of the following is not a recognised risk factor for early atherosclerosis**
    A. Homocystinuria
    B. Hyperthyroidism
    C. Pseudoxanthoma elasticum
    D. Nephrotic syndrome

134. **Which of the following is least important cause of dissection of aorta**
    A. Arteriosclerosis
    B. Coarctation of aorta
    C. Marfan's syndrome
    D. Pregnancy

135. **Which enzyme rises earliest in AMI**
    A. SGPT
    B. LDH
    C. SCOT
    D. CPK

Ans: 127-A 128-C 129-D 130-C 131-C 132-B 133-B 134-A 135-D

136. Which of the following is not a side effect of amiodarone
    A. Photosensitivity
    B. Hepatitis
    C. Tachyarrhythmias
    D. Alveolitis

137. Syncopal attack is associated with all of the following *except*
    A. Myocarditis
    B. Hypertrophic cardiomyopathy
    C. Ventricular fibrillation
    D. Aortic stenosis

138. Compression of the feeding artery abruptly reduces the heart rate in arteriovenous fistula, and is known as
    A. Tinel's sign
    B. Hoover sign
    C. Bing sign
    D. Branham's sign

139. Pulmonary regurgitation is never associated with
    A. Pulmonary fibrosis
    B. Pulmonary oedema
    C. Pulmonary hypertension
    D. Obstructive mitral valve disease

140. Hypocalcaemia arrests the heart in
    A. Mid-systole
    B. Diastole
    C. Mid-diastole
    D. Systole

141. The drug contraindicated in pregnancy-induced hypertension is
    A. Hydralazine
    B. Enalapril
    C. Methyldopa
    D. Labetalol

142. Reversed splitting of S_2 is found in
    A. LBBB
    B. RBBB
    C. Left ventricular pacing
    D. Aortic regurgitation

143. All of the following drugs may be used in congestive cardiac failure *except*
    A. Spironolactone
    B. Bucindolol
    C. Propranolol
    D. Digoxin

144. Janeway's spot in SBE is found in
    A. Palms
    B. Fundus
    C. Nailbed
    D. Palate

145. Pulsus bisferiens is best perceived in
    A. Radial
    B. Brachial
    C. Femoral
    D. Any of the above

Ans: 136-C 137-A 138-D 139-B 140-B 141-B 142-A 143-C 144-A 145-B

146. Which of the following cardioselective beta-blockers is used in heart failure
    A. Carvedilol   B. Atenolol
    C. Labetalol   D. Pindolol

147. Which one is false regarding the presence of ejection click
    A. Occurs immediately after S_1
    B. Stenosis is severe
    C. Presence indicates stenosis at valvular level
    D. Sharp and high-pitched clicking sound

148 Congestive cardiac failure may be seen in all *except*
    A. Fallot's tetralogy   B. MS
    C. PDA   D. Coarctation of aorta

149. Treatment by heparin is best monitored by
    A. Prothrombin time (PT)
    B. Clotting time (CT)
    C. Activated partial thromboplastin time (APTT)
    D. Fibrin degradation product (FDP)

150. Major cardiovascular manifestation in cri-du-chat syndrome is
    A. Bicuspid aortic valve   B. VSD
    C. PDA   D. Dextrocardia

151. 'Nitrate tolerance' developing as a result of treating ischaemic heart disease by mononitrates is prevented by
    A. Twice daily dosage schedule B. Night-time single dosage
    C. Eccentric dosage schedule   D. Morning-time single dosage

152. All of the following may produce hemiplegia by cerebral embolism *except*
    A. Mitral valve prolapse
    B. Atrial fibrillation
    C. Subacute bacterial endocarditis
    D. Right atrial myxoma

153. Drug of choice in acute management of PSVT is
    A. Amiodarone   B. Verapramil
    C. Metoprolol   D. Adenosine

154. Which of the following gives rise to pulsation at the back
    A. Coarctation of aorta   B. Budd-Chiari syndrome
    C. Hyperkinetic circulatory states D. Aortic aneurysm

Ans: 146-A 147-B 148-A 149-A 150-B 151-C 152-D 153-D 154-A

155. **'Absolute' contraindication of thrombolytic therapy in AMI is**
    A. Severe menstrual bleeding   B. Bacterial endocarditis
    C. H/O intraocular bleeeding   D. Pregnancy

156. **Propranolol can be used in all *except***
    A. Systemic hypertension
    B. Congestive cardiac failure
    C. Angina pectoris
    D. Supraventricular tachyarrhythmias

157. **Heart valve commonly affected in IV drug abusers is**
    A. Pulmonary valve   B. Mitral valve
    C. Tricuspid valve   D. Aortic valve

158. **Which is not an example of vasospastic disorder**
    A. Livedo reticularis   B. Acrocyanosis
    C. Raynaud's phenomenon   D. Deep vein thrombosis

159. **In right ventricular myocardial infarction, which of the following additional therapies is needed**
    A. Diuretics   B. Calcium gluconate
    C. IV fluid   D. Restriction of fluid

160. **Ventricular fibrillation is best treated by**
    A. IV amiodarone   B. Carotid massage
    C. Electrical cardioversion   D. IV lignocaine

161. **All of the following are characteristics of right ventricular infarction *except***
    A. Increased JVP   B. Pulmonary congestion
    C. Hypotension   D. Kussmaul's sign

162. **P-wave in ECG is absent in**
    A. Atrial fibrillation   B. Atrial flutter
    C. Hypokalaemia   D. PSVT

163. **Ibutilide is an antiarrhythmic agent of**
    A. Class I   B. Class II
    C. Class III   D. Class IV

164. **Verapamil is indicated in all *except***
    A. Atrial fibrillation   B. Acute left ventricular failure
    C. Supraventricular tachycardia D. Angina pectoris

Ans: 155-D 156-B 157-C 158-D 159-C 160-C 161-B 162-A 163-C 164-B

165. **Arteriovenous fistula is associated with**
   A. Sinus tachycardia   B. Sinus bradycardia
   C. Hypotension   D. Low pulse pressure

166. **Hyperthyroid heart disease is manifested by**
   A. Pericardial effusion   B. Diminished cardiac output
   C. Prolonged circulation time D. Paroxysmal atrial fibrillation

167. **Earliest valvular lesion in acute rheumatic carditis is**
   A. MS   B. AI
   C. MI   D. AS

168. **Which of the following drugs raises HDL cholesterol**
   A. Nicotinic acid   B. Gemfibrozil
   C. Probucol   D. Lovastatin

169. **Pedal pulse is 'absent' in all *except***
   A. Buerger's disease   B. Leriche's syndrome
   C. Coarctation of aorta   D. Peripheral embolism

170. **The ECG finding in hypercalcaemia is**
   A. Shortened PR interval   B. Tall T-waves
   C. Diminished QT interval D. Increased PR interval

171. **'Hilar dance' is characteristic of**
   A. ASD   B. VSD
   C. PDA   D. Transposition of great vessels

172. **In coarctation of aorta, rib notching is seen in**
   A. 3–6th rib   B. 6–9th rib
   C. 10–12th rib   D. 1–12th rib

173. **Dressler's syndrome results from**
   A. Bacteria   B. Autoimmune reaction
   C. Virus   D. Protozoa

174. **A$_2$ in aortic stenosis is characteristically**
   A. Diminished   B. Ringing in character
   C. Normal in character D. Accentuated

175. **Which of the following is present in most of the patients of SBE**
   A. Murmur   B. Osler's node
   C. Clubbing   D. Splenomegaly

Ans: 165-A 166-D 167-C 168-A 169-C 170-C 171-A 172-B 173-B 174-A 175-A

176. When a patient of unstable angina worsens by nitroglycerine, the diagnosis is
    A. MS
    B. Left main coronary artery stenosis
    C. MI
    D. Idiopathic subaortic stenosis

177. Increased PR interval is observed in
    A. AV nodal rhythm   B. First degee heart block
    C. W-P-W syndrome   D. Low atrial rhythm

178. Pulmonary capillary wedge pressure is increased in all *except*
    A. Right ventricular infarction
    B. Cardiac tamponade
    C. Acute mitral regurgitation
    D. Cardiogenic shock due to myocardial dysfunction

179. Which of the following does not produce continuous murmur over the chest
    A. Ruptured sinus of Valsalva   B. Patent ductus arteriosus
    C. Aortopulmonary window   D. Ventricular septal defect

180. Inverted P-wave in lead I, upright P-wave in aVR and gradual diminution of the height of R-waves in precordial leads are found in
    A. Emphysema
    B. Faulty interchange of right and left arm electrode
    C. Dextrocardia
    D. ECG taken at height of deep inspiration

181. Commonest cause of displacement of apex beat is
    A. Left ventricular hypertrophy B. Thoracic deformity
    C. Cardiomyopathy   D. Right ventricular hypertrophy

182. Graham Steell murmur is found in
    A. Severe pulmonary hypertension
    B. Subacute bacterial endocarditis
    C. Idiopathic hypertrophic subaortic stenosis (IHSS)
    D. Tricuspid atresia

183. Drug to be avoided in hypertensive encephalopathy
    A. Labetalol   B. Diazoxide
    C. Methyldopa   D. Sodium nitroprusside

Ans: 176-D 177-B 178-A 179-D 180-C 181-B 182-A 183-C

184. **High-volume double-peaked pulse is found in all *except***
    A. AI
    B. IHSS
    C. AS with AI
    D. MI

185. **Boot-shaped heart with oilgaemic lung fields is found in**
    A. ASD
    B. Tetralogy of Fallot
    C. Coarctation of aorta
    D. Transposition of great vessels

186. **Exercise tolerance test (TMT) is absolutely contraindicated in**
    A. Aortic stenosis
    B. Buerger's disease
    C. Unstable angina
    D. Coarctation of aorta

187. **Osler's node is classically seen in**
    A. Libman-Sacks endocarditis
    B. Marantic endocarditis
    C. Acute staphylococcal endocarditis
    D. *Candida albicans* endocarditis

188. **Commonest aetiology of tricuspid incompetence in clinical practice is**
    A. Endocarditis of IV drug abusers
    B. Rheumatic heart disease
    C. Right ventricular dilatation
    D. Collagen vascular disease

189. **Commonest heart valve abnormality revealed after AMI is**
    A. AI
    B. MI
    C. AS
    D. MS

190. **Which of the following heart sounds occurs shortly after S_1**
    A. Ejection click
    B. Opening snap
    C. Tumour plop in atrial myxoma
    D. Pericardial knock

191. **Which of the following is not a natural vasodilator**
    A. Bradykinin
    B. Histamine
    C. Endothelin
    D. Nitric oxide

192. **Pseudoclaudication is due to compression of**
    A. Inferior vena cava
    B. Cauda equina
    C. Femoral artery
    D. Popliteal artery

Ans: 184-D 185-B 186-A 187-C 188-C 189-B 190-A 191-C 192-B

193. **The chance of SBE is lowest in**
   A. VSD
   B. MS
   C. AI
   D. PDA

194. **Increased level of which of the following is not a risk factor for IHD**
   A. Homocysteine
   B. PAI-I
   C. Transferrin
   D. Lipoprotein

195. **Which is not included in 'lipid tetrad' in risk factors for coronary heart disease**
   A. ↑ VLDL
   B. ↓ HDL
   C. ↑ Small dense LDL
   D. ↑ Lipoprotein (a)

196. **Regarding ischaemic heart disease (IHD) in India, which of the following is not true**
   A. High incidence of insulin resistance
   B. Prevalence of CAD is more in India in comparison to developed countries
   C. Occurs a decade earlier
   D. High LDL in Indian population

197. **Which is not a predisposing factor to dissecting aneurysm of aorta**
   A. Pregnancy
   B. Syphilitic aortitis
   C. Systemic hypertension
   D. Marfan's syndrome

198. **Acute pericarditis is a 'recognised' complication of all *except***
   A. Acute pancreatitis
   B. Chronic renal failure
   C. Systemic lupus erythematosus
   D. Gonorrhoea

199. **Coronary atherosclerosis is not linked to**
   A. *H. pylori*
   B. Cytomegalovirus
   C. HIV
   D. *Chlamydia*

200. **Which of the following is false regarding complete heart block**
   A. Low-volume pulse
   B. Irregular cannon waves in neck vein
   C. Regular pulse rate
   D. Beat to beat variation of blood pressure

Ans: 193-B 194-C 195-A 196-D 197-B 198-A 199-C 200-A

201. **In a patient with MS in sinus rhythm, severity of lesion is indicated by**
    A. Late and loud opening snap
    B. Presence of S_3
    C. Graham Steell murmur
    D. Harshness of mid-diastolic murmur

202. **Tall R-wave in lead V_1 of the ECG is characteristic of**
    A. Hypokalaemia
    B. Left ventricular hypertrophy
    C. True posterior myocardial infarction
    D. Left bundle branch block

203. **Right axis deviation in ECG is found in**
    A. Ostium primum type ASD   B. W-P-W syndrome
    C. Hyperkalaemia   D. During inspiration

204. **Pregnancy-associated hypertension should not be treated with**
    A. Labetalol   B. Telmisartan
    C. α-methyldopa   D. Amlodipine

205. **Still's murmur is**
    A. Associated with thrill   B. Best heard over mitral area
    C. Usually diastolic in timing   D. Commonly found in children

206. **Murmur of hypertrophic obstructive cardiomyopathy is decreased by**
    A. Leg raising   B. Valsalva manoeuvre
    C. Amyl nitrite inhalation   D. Standing

207. **Accelerated hypertension should not have**
    A. Retinal haemorrhage   B. Arteriovenous nipping
    C. 'Silver-wire' arteries   D. Papilloedema

208. **Clinically, commonest type of shock is**
    A. Neurogenic   B. Cardiogenic
    C. Septic   D. Hypovolaemic

209. **XXXXX-karyotype is usually associated with**
    A. VSD   B. PDA
    C. ASD   D. Dextrocardia

210. **When given once daily in prevention of IHD, aspirin has halflife of**
    A. 20 minutes   B. 1 hour
    C. 6 hours   D. 24 hours

Ans: 201-C 202-C 203-D 204-B 205-D 206-A 207-D 208-D 209-B 210-A

211. **Angio-oedema is not uncommon in treatment with**
    A. Amrinone
    B. Amlodipine
    C. Lisinopril
    D. Amiodarone

212. **Syphilis may give rise to**
    A. Berry aneurysm
    B. Coronary osteal stenosis
    C. Pulmonary stenosis
    D. Aneurysm of abdominal aorta

213. **JVP is usually increased in**
    A. Cardiogenic shock
    B. Hypovolaemic shock
    C. Anaphylactic shock
    D. Septic shock

214. **Still's murmur is**
    A. Systolic innocent murmur
    B. Early diastolic murmur of pulmonary regurgitation
    C. Harsh systolic murmur in thyrotoxicosis
    D. Systolic murmur in complete heart block

215. **Commonest congenital cyanotic heart disease with cyanosis at birth is**
    A. Transposition of great vessels
    B. Tricuspid atresia
    C. Fallot's tetralogy
    D. Ebstein's anomaly

216. **Cri-du-chat syndrome does not have**
    A. VSD
    B. Cat-like cry
    C. Deletion of short arm of chromosome 5
    D. Mongoloid slant of eyes

217. **Jug-handle apprearance in chest X-ray is characteristic of**
    A. Tricuspid atresia
    B. Primary pulmonary hypertension
    C. Transposition of great vessels
    D. Constrictive pericarditis

218. **Negative 'acute phase reactant' is**
    A. Platelets
    B. Alkaline phosphatase
    C. Uric acid
    D. LDH

Ans: 211-C 212-B 213-A 214-A 215-A 216-D 217-B 218-C

219. Cardiac anomalies associated with tetralogy of Fallot are all *except*

    A. Right-sided aortic arch
    B. Persistent right-sided SVC
    C. Aortic regurgitation
    D. PDA

220. Holt-Oram syndrome is characterized by

    A. Fingerisation of thumb   B. Absent clavicle
    C. VSD   D. Asplenia

221. Which is true in 'maladie de Roger'

    A. Moderate VSD
    B. Haemodynamically significant
    C. Thrill and pansystolic murmur are very prominent
    D. A small fraction closes by the year 10

222. PDA is life saving in all of the following *except*

    A. Hypoplastic left heart syndrome
    B. Pulmonary atresia
    C. Severe coarctation of aorta
    D. Total anomalous pulmonary venous connection

223. Eisenmenger's syndrome should not have

    A. Wide split of S_2 with loud P_2
    B. Central cyanosis
    C. Pansystolic murmur of tricuspid incompetence
    D. Prominent a-wave in neck veins

224. Familial myxomas may be a part of syndrome complex with endocrine overactivity like

    A. Hyperthyroidism
    B. Cushing's syndrome
    C. Hyperparathyroidism
    D. Phaeochromocytoma

Ans: 219-B   220-A   221-C   222-D   223-A   224-B

4

Pulmonology

1. Clubbing is present in all *except*
   - A. Fibrosing alveolitis
   - B. Cystic fibrosis
   - C. Emphysema
   - D. Lung abscess

2. Which is false regarding transudative pleural effusion
   - A. Protein < 3.0 g/100 ml
   - B. Pleural fluid/serum LDH ratio <0.6
   - C. pH<7.2
   - D. Specific gravity <1.016

3. Which is an example of exudative pleural effusion
   - A. Nephrotic syndrome
   - B. Constrictive pericarditis
   - C. SVC syndrome
   - D. Rheumatoid arthritis

4. Commonest cause of hypertrophic osteoarthropathy is
   - A. Fallot's tetralogy
   - B. Bronchiectasis
   - C. Mesothelioma of pleura
   - D. Bronchogenic carcinoma

5. Which of the following drugs may produce pleural effusion
   - A. Losartan
   - B. Miltefosine
   - C. Amiodarone
   - D. Propranolol

6. All are causes of pseudoclubbing *except*
   - A. Leprosy
   - B. Ulcerative colitis
   - C. Acromegaly
   - D. Scleroderma

7. Bilateral pleural effusion is commonly seen in
   - A. SLE
   - B. Nephrotic syndrome
   - C. Pulmonary tuberculosis
   - D. Congestive cardiac failure

8. Lovibond's angle is approximately
   - A. 120°
   - B. 140°
   - C. 160°
   - D. 175°

Ans: 1-C 2-C 3-D 4-D 5-C 6-B 7-A 8-C

9. **Haemorrhagic pleural effusion may be seen in**
   A. Cirrhosis of liver
   B. Pulmonary tuberculosis
   C. SLE
   D. Myxoedema

10. **Worldwide commonest cause of haemoptysis is**
    A. Pulmonary tuberculosis
    B. Bronchogenic carcinoma
    C. Chronic bronchitis
    D. Pneumonia

11. **Woody dullness in precussion over chest is classically found in**
    A. Thickened pleura
    B. Consolidation
    C. Collapse of the lung
    D. Pleural effusion

12. **All are examples of "honeycomb lung' *except***
    A. Tuberous sclerosis
    B. Scleroderma
    C. Lung abscess
    D. Bronchiectasis

13. **Pleural rub is characteristically**
    A. Uniphasic
    B. Superficial, scratchy
    C. Alters with coughing
    D. Never palpable

14. **Cheyne-Stokes respiration is classically seen in all *except***
    A. Hepatocellular failure
    B. Uraemia
    C. Opium poisoning
    D. Raised intracranial tension

15. **Convulsions may be produced by all of the antituberculous drugs *except***
    A. Ciprofloxacin
    B. Prothionamide
    C. INH
    D. Cycloserine

16. **Bronchial breath sound is found in all *except***
    A. Collapse with patent bronchus
    B. Bronchial asthma
    C. Superficial, big, empty cavity with patent bronchus
    D. Bronchopleural fistula

17. **Aegophony may be found in**
    A. Pneumothorax
    B. Emphysema
    C. Consolidation
    D. Superficial, empty cavity

18. **Typical cadence of tachycardia, overshoot of BP and bradycardia after Valsalva manoeuvre is found in all *except***
    A. ASD
    B. Ischaemic heart disease
    C. Bronchial asthma
    D. Pleural effusion

Ans: 9-B 10-C 11-B 12-C 13-B 14-A 15-B 16-B 17-C 18-A

19. **In a patient of consolidation, which one of the following is increased commonly**

    A. Myotactic irritability
    B. Vocal fremitus
    C. Rhonchial fremitus
    D. Palpable coarse crepitations

20. **Platypnoea may be found in**

    A. COPD
    B. Acute severe asthma
    C. Pneumonia
    D. Selective paralysis of intercostal muscles

21. **Loss of Traube's space tympanicity is found in all *except***

    A. Splenic rupture
    B. Achalasia cardia
    C. Ca. of fundus of stomach
    D. Pericardial effusion

22. **Restriction of bilateral chest movement is found in all *except***

    A. Myasthenia gravis
    B. Ankylosing spondylitis
    C. Viperide snake bite
    D. Diffuse interstitial fibrosis

23. **Crepitations uninfluenced by coughing are found in**

    A. Acute pulmonary oedema
    B. Consolidation
    C. Fibrosing alveolitis
    D. Lung abscess

24. **Pink, frothy and profuse sputum is seen in**

    A. Pneumoconiosis
    B. Lobar pneumonia
    C. Acute pulmonary oedema
    D. Aspergilloma

25. **Bilateral hypertranslucency in chest X-ray (PA view) is seen in all *except***

    A. Emphysema
    B. Under-exposed film
    C. Multiple bullae
    D. Fallot's tetralogy with pulmonary atresia

26. **Pneumatocele is found in pneumonia caused by**

    A. *Staphylococcus aureus*
    B. *Klebsiella preumoniae*
    C. *Streptococcus preumoniae*
    D. *Mycoplasma preumoniae*

27. **In performing a chest X-ray (PA view), the tube-film distance should be**

    A. 2 feet
    B. 4 feet
    C. 6 feet
    D. 8 feet

28. **Non-cardiogenic pulmonary oedema is seen in all *except***

    A. Fulminant hepatic failure
    B. Haemorrhagic pancreatitis
    C. Deep sea diving
    D. Malignant malaria

Ans: 19-B 20-D 21-D 22-C 23-C 24-C 25-B 26-A 27-C 28-C

29. **P-pulmonale in EGG is seen in**

    A. Hydropneumothorax
    B. Chronic cor pulmonale
    C. Pulmonary tuberculosis
    D. Allergic bronchopulmonary aspergillosis

30. **Amphoric breath sound is found in**

    A. Pleural effusion
    B. Superficial, big empty cavity in lung
    C. Consolidation
    D. Open pneumothorax

31. **The lower part of right border of cardiac silhouette in a chest X-ray (PA view) is usually formed by**

    A. Right atrium
    B. Inferior vena cava
    C. Right ventricle
    D. Superior vena cava

32. **A patient with haemoptysis and having depressed bridge of the nose is diagnostic of**

    A. Rickets
    B. Wegener's granulomatosis
    C. Congenital syphilis
    D. Rhinocerebral mucormycosis

33. **Low voltage in EGG is seen in**

    A. Thin chest wall
    B. Consolidation
    C. Hyperthyroidism
    D. Emphysema

34. **Which of the following is false regarding 'aging'**

    A. Fall in vital capacity
    B. Increase in functional residual capacity
    C. Fall in residual volume
    D. Increase in closing volume

35. **Diffusing capacity of lung at rest is**

    A. 5 (ml/min)/mm Hg
    B. 20 (ml/min)/mm Hg
    C. 35 (ml/min)/mm Hg
    D. 55 (ml/min)/mm Hg

36. **The elastic recoil of lung is severely diminished in**

    A. Chronic bronchitis
    B. Emphysema
    C. Bronchogenic carcinoma
    D. Bronchial asthma

37. **Rib notching exclusively in the lower border is seen in**

    A. Neurofibromatosis
    B. Hyperparathyroidism
    C. Coarctation of aorta
    D. Pulmonary stenosis

Ans: 29-B 30-D 31-A 32-B 33-D 34-C 35-B 36-B 37-C

38. 'Closing volume' of the lung is increased in
    A. Cigarette smoking   B. Obesity
    C. Anaemia   D. Bronchiectasis

39. Bilateral hilar lymphadenopathy is seen in all *except*
    A. Sarcoidosis
    B. Bronchogenic carcinoma
    C. Pneumoconiosis
    D. Lymphoma

40. Impairment of diffusion is seen in all *except*
    A. Sarcoidosis   B. Pleural mesothelioma
    C. Emphysema   D. Anaemia

41. Melanoptysis (black sputum) is seen in
    A. Coal worker's pneumoconiosis
    B. Ochronosis
    C. Maple syrup urine disease
    D. Goodpasture's disease

42. Reduced compliance of lung is seen in all *except*
    A. Diffuse interstitial fibrosis   B. Atelectasis
    C. Left ventricular failure   D. Emphysema

43. Which one of the following is not a paraneoplastic syndrome in bronchogenic carcinoma
    A. Cachexia   B. Haemoptysis
    C. Polymyositis   D. SIADH

44. Physiologic dead space is increased in all *except*
    A. Pulmonary thromboembolism
    B. Diffuse interstitial fibrosis
    C. COPD
    D. Pulmonary tuberculosis

45. Regarding hypoventilation, all are true *except*
    A. Occurs in severe kyphoscoliosis
    B. Hypoxaemia
    C. Hypercapnia
    D. Hypoxaemia is not corrected by 100% O_2

46. All of the following are restrictive lung diseases *except*
    A. Sarcoidosis   B. Cystic fibrosis
    C. Myasthenia gravis   D. Obesity

Ans: 38-A 39-C 40-B 41-A 42-D 43-B 44-D 45-D 46-B

47. 'Monday dyspnoea' is classically described in

    A. Byssinosis   B. Bagassosis
    C. Silicosis   D. Coal worker's pneumoconiosis

48. Farmer's lung is caused by

    A. Sugarcane fibres   B. *Micropolyspora faeni*
    C. *Bacillus subtilis*   D. Isocyanates

49. All of the following may aggravate bronchial asthma *except*

    A. Pituitary snuff   B. Acetylsalicylic acid
    C. β-blockers   D. Sodium salicylate

50. Drug-induced eosinophilic pneumonia is caused by all *except*

    A. Penicillins   B. Nitrofurantoin
    C. Chlorpropamide   D. Hydrochlorthiazides

51. Which of the following is not an example of hypersensitivity pneumonitis

    A. Bagassosis   B. Byssinosis
    C. Farmer's lung   D. Maple bark disease

52. Impaired diffusion of lung characteristically produces

    A. Hypercapnia
    B. Rarely develops hypoxaemia
    C. Severe hypercapnia on exercise
    D. No relief after 100% O_2 inhalation

53. Allergic bronchopulmonary aspergillosis occurs in

    A. Pulmonary tuberculous cavity   B. Cystic lesion of sarcoid
    C. Atopic asthmatic person   D. In immunocompromised host

54. Which of the following does not belong to the triad of symptomatic bronchial asthma

    A. Chest pain   B. Dyspnoea
    C. Wheeze   D. Cough

55. Malt worker's lung is caused by

    A. *Cryptostroma corticate*   B. *Thermoactinomyces vulgaris*
    C. *Streptomyces olivaceus*   D. *Aspergillus clavatus*

56. Caplan's syndrome is coal worker's pneumoconiosis associated with

    A. SLE   B. Scleroderma
    C. Rheumatoid arthritis   D. Ankylosing spondylitis

Ans: 47-A 48-B 49-D 50-D 51-B 52-B 53-C 54-A 55-D 56-C

57. In lobar pneumonia, which of the following is true in arterial blood

    A. $\downarrow$ Po$_2$ and $\uparrow$ Pco$_2$ B. $\downarrow$ Po$_2$ and $\downarrow$ Pco$_2$
    C. $\downarrow$ Po$_2$ and normal Pco$_2$ D. Normal Po$_2$ and $\uparrow$ Pco$_2$

58. Viral pneumonia may have

    A. Signs of consolidation in chest
    B. Splenomegaly
    C. High WBC count
    D. Foul-smelling expectoration

59. Which one of the following is false in silicosis

    A. Predominant involvement of lower lobes
    B. Develops into progressive massive fibrosis
    C. Predisposes to infection by *Mycobacterium tuberculosis*
    D. Hilar nodes may show 'eggshell' calcification

60. All are commonly seen in Legionella pneumophila-induced pneumonia *except*

    A. Cavitation   B. Hyponatraemia
    C. Proteinuria   D. Confusion

61. Chest X-ray shows miliary mottlings in all *except*

    A. Extrinsic allergic alveolitis   B. Chickenpox pneumonia
    C. Tuberous sclerosis   D. Pulmonary haemosiderosis

62. In lobar pneumonia, which is not true

    A. Trachea deviated to the opposite side
    B. Woody dullness on percussion
    C. Tubular breath sound
    D. Presence of whispering pectoriloquy

63. Asbestosis is not related to

    A. Mesothelioma of peritoneum
    B. Carcinoma of the lung
    C. Progressive massive fibrosis
    D. Mesothelioma of pleura

64. Which of the following is false regarding indications of hospitalisation in pneumonia

    A. Respiratory rate >30/min with dyspnoea
    B. Temperature >103°F
    C. Pulse rate >140 beats/min
    D. Signs of meningism

Ans: 57-B 58-B 59-A 60-A 61-C 62-A 63-C 64-B

65. Characteristic of *Mycoplasma pneumoniae*-pneumonia are all *except*
    A. Headache
    B. Non-productive cough
    C. Pleural effusion
    D. Bullous myringitis

66. Which of the following is sex-linked disease
    A. Yellow nail syndrome
    B. Cystic fibrosis
    C. Lesch-Nyhan syndrome
    D. Polycystic kidney

67. Expectoration of chalky sediments with gritty particles are diagnostic of
    A. Bronchorrhoea
    B. Pulmonary alveolar proteinosis
    C. Melanoptysis
    D. Broncholithiasis

68. Broncholithiasis is usually late complication of some infections; which does not fall in this group
    A. Histoplasmosis
    B. Tuberculosis
    C. Coccidioidomycosis
    D. Aspergillosis

69. Which is true in a predominant "blue bloater"
    A. Vital capacity is markedly diminished
    B. H/O repeated episodes of respiratory insufficiency
    C. Elastic recoil is much diminished
    D. Pulmonary hypertension does not complicate the disease

70. Most predominant infective agent of respiratory tract in cystic fibrosis is
    A. *Staphylococcus aureus*
    B. *Pseudomonas aeruginosa*
    C. *Escherichia coli*
    D. Anaerobes

71. In chronic bronchitis, the Reid index should be
    A. >0.20
    B. >0.34
    C. >0.38
    D. >0.52

72. Which is not a part of 'Kartagener's syndrome'
    A. Dextrocardia
    B. Sinusitis
    C. Impotence
    D. Bronchiectasis

73. Which is false regarding emphysema
    A. Pao_2 65–75 mm Hg
    B. Increaesd diffusion capacity
    C. $Paco_2$ 35–40 mm Hg
    D. Decreased elastic recoil

74. Which is not a recognised complication of cystic fibrosis
    A. Atelectasis
    B. Bronchiectasis
    C. Pleural effusion
    D. Pulmonary hypertension

Ans: 65-C 66-C 67-D 68-D 69-B 70-B 71-D 72-C 73-B 74-C

75. Which of the following is not common in primary pulmonary tuberculosis

    A. Cavity   B. Fibrosis
    C. Lymphadenopathy   D. Pleural effusion

76. Which of the following is not a bedside feature of fibrosing alveolitis

    A. Orthopnoea   B. Anaemia
    C. Clubbing   D. Velcro crepitations

77. Chronic respiratory failure is not seen in

    A. Diffuse interstitial fibrosis   B. Emphysema
    C. Pneumothorax   D. Chronic bronchitis

78. Commonest middle mediastinal mass is

    A. Lymphoma   B. Aortic aneurysm
    C. Bronchogenic cyst   D. Thymoma

79. Which of the following is not associated with interstitial lung disease

    A. Graft versus host disease
    B. Idiopathic pulmonary haemosiderosis
    C. Bronchiectasis
    D. Scleroderma

80. Commonest posterior mediastinal tumour is

    A. Neurofibroma   B. Lymphoma
    C. Teratodermoid   D. Metastatic carcinoma

81. All of the following drugs may produce fibrosing alveolitis *except*

    A. Busulfan   B. Bleomycin
    C. Beclomethasone   D. Nitrofuratoin

82. Lung abscess is not a complication of

    A. Malignancy
    B. Bronchopneumonia
    C. Wegener's granulomatosis
    D. Suppurative staphylococcal pneumonia

83. Bilateral parotid enlargement is seen in all *except*

    A. Sjögren's syndrome   B. Guanethidine-induced
    C. Sarcoidosis   D. Guillain-Barré syndrome

84. Silo-filler's disease is inhalation of

    A. Nitrogen dioxide   B. Hydrogen fluoride
    C. Sulphur dioxide   D. Chlorine

Ans: 75-A 76-B 77-C 78-B 79-C 80-A 81-C 82-B 83-D 84-A

85. α₁-antitrypsin deficiency PiZZ type have predominant

    A. Paraseptal emphysema
    B. Centriacinar emphysema
    C. Paracicatrical emphysema
    D. Panacinar emphysema

86. Which opportunistic organism commonly affects patients of pulmonary alveolar proteinosis

    A. *Pseudomonas*
    B. *Staphylococcus*
    C. *Pneumococcus*
    D. *Nocardia*

87. Bronchopleural fistula is commonly due to

    A. Pulmonary tuberculosis
    B. Bronchogenic carcinoma
    C. Lung cyst
    D. Honeycomb lung

88. The most reliable symptom of acute pulmonary thromboembolism is

    A. Substernal chest pain
    B. Haemoptysis
    C. Breathlessness
    D. Syncope

89. Which of the following is false regarding Pickwickian syndrome

    A. Marked obesity
    B. Hyperventilation
    C. Somnolence
    D. Right-sided heart failure

90. The commonest benign pulmonary neoplasm is

    A. Adenoma
    B. Lipoma
    C. Hamartoma
    D. Fibroma

91. Large amount of eosinophils in the sputum is diagnostic of

    A. Staphylococcal pneumonia
    B. Fibrosing alveolitis
    C. Pulmonary aspergillosis
    D. Cystic fibrosis

92. Commonest histologic variety of bronchogenic carcinoma is

    A. Small cell carcinoma
    B. Large cell carcinoma
    C. Epidermoid carcinoma
    D. Adenocarcinoma

93. Which of the following is false regarding primary pulmonary hypertension

    A. Age ranges 20–40 yrs
    B. Females are the main victims
    C. Primarily due to heart disease
    D. Calcium channel blockers may alleviate symptoms

94. Investigation of highest diagnostic efficacy in acute pulmonary thromboembolism is

    A. ECG
    B. Arterial blood gas estimation
    C. Contrast-enhanced spiral CT scan
    D. Ventilation-perfusion lung scans

Ans: 85-D 86-D 87-A 88-C 89-B 90-A 91-C 92-C 93-C 94-D

95. A high amylase in pleural fluid is found in all *except*
    A. Oesophageal rupture
    B. Bronchogenic carcinoma
    C. Sarcoidosis
    D. Acute pancreatitis

96. Laennec's pearls and Curschmann's spirals in sputum are characteristically seen in
    A. Pulmonary tuberculosis
    B. Farmer's lung
    C. Chronic bronchitis
    D. Bronchial asthma

97. Which of the following is not a neurological paraneoplastic syndrome of bronchogenic carcinoma
    A. Eaton-Lambert syndrome
    B. Cerebral thrombosis
    C. Retinal blindness
    D. Subacute cerebellar degeneration

98. Thymoma may be associated with all *except*
    A. AIDS
    B. Pure red cell aplasia
    C. Cushing's syndrome
    D. Myasthenia gravis

99. Which of the following is not in the list of bedside severity assessment of bronchial asthma
    A. Kussmaul's sign
    B. Pulsus paradoxus
    C. Silent chest
    D. Central cyanosis

100. Which of the following is used to treat cystic fibrosis
    A. Low-molecular weight heparin
    B. High dose of glucocorticoids
    C. Dornase alfa
    D. Zafirlukast

101. Pure O_2 therapy may produce all of the following *except*
    A. Acute lung injury
    B. Respiratory depression
    C. Fibrosis of the lung
    D. Consolidation of the lung

102. Brassy cough is seen in
    A. Recurrent laryngeal nerve palsy
    B. Acute laryngitis
    C. Heavy smokers
    D. Carcinoma of the larynx

103. Therapy in idiopathic pulmonary fibrosis includes all *except*
    A. Colchicine
    B. Cyclophosphamide
    C. Interferon-gamma
    D. Prednisolone

104. Upper border of liver dullness is elevated in all *except*
    A. Ascites
    B. Subdiaphragmatic abscess (right)
    C. Pneumothorax (right)
    D. Pleural effusion (right)

Ans: 95-C 96-D 97-B 98-A 99-A 100-C 101-C 102-D 103-C 104-C

105. **Commonest cause of respiratory failure is**
    A. Emphysema
    B. Fibrosing alveolitis
    C. Bronchial asthma
    D. Chronic bronchitis

106. **All are true in pneumomediastinum** *except*
    A. May occur during an attack of asthma
    B. Acute mediastinitis is a sequela
    C. Amphoric breath sound in auscultation
    D. Presence of Hamman's sign

107. **Acute lung injury (ARDS) should be differentiated from**
    A. Acute LVF
    B. Congestive cardiac failure
    C. Acute severe asthma
    D. Spontaneous pneumothorax

108. **Stridor is characteristically found in**
    A. Tropical eosinophilia
    B. Laryngeal diphtheria
    C. Carcinoid syndrome
    D. Cardiac asthma

109. **All are features of hypercapnia** *except*
    A. Capillary pulsation
    B. Central cyanosis
    C. Papilloedema
    D. Asterixis

110. **Serum angiotensin-converting enzyme (ACE) level is increased in all** *except*
    A. Sarcoidosis
    B. Primary biliary cirrhosis
    C. Asbestosis
    D. Silicosis

111. **Hyperbaric oxygen therapy is indicated in all** *except*
    A. Crush injury
    B. Decompression sickness
    C. Acute osteomyelitis
    D. Carbon monoxide poisoning

112. **The dome of diaphragm is elevated in**
    A. Emphysema
    B. Pleural effusion
    C. Cirrhosis of liver
    D. Diaphragmatic palsy

113. **Classic dermatological manifestation of chronic sarcoidosis is**
    A. Erythema nodosum
    B. Maculopapular rash
    C. Lupus pernio
    D. Subcutaneous nodules

114. **Commonest cause of superior mediastinal syndrome is**
    A. Lymphoma
    B. Thymoma
    C. Bronchogenic carcinoma
    D. Retrosternal goitre

Ans: 105-D 106-C 107-A 108-B 109-B 110-B 111-C 112-D 113-C 114-C

115. **Pulmonary fibrosis is not produced by**
    A. Tuberculosis
    B. Cor pulmonale
    C. Progressive systemic sclerosis
    D. Rheumatoid arthritis

116. **Cranial nerve most commonly affected in sarcoidosis is**
    A. VIIth
    B. IInd
    C. Vth
    D. Xth

117. **Commonest cause of death in sarcoidosis is**
    A. Cor pulmonale
    B. Pneumonia
    C. Nephrocalcinosis
    D. Neurosarcoidosis

118. **Regarding diaphragmatic palsy, which is false**
    A. Bilateral palsy is commoner than unilateral palsy
    B. Paradoxical respiration
    C. Positive sniff test
    D. Tachypnoea

119. **Reactivation of pulmonary tuberculosis is due to**
    A. Malnutrition
    B. Low perfusion
    C. High ventilation
    D. Low Pao_2

120. **All of the following are allergic reactions to tuberculosis** *except*
    A. Few cases of pleural effusion
    B. Erythema nodosum
    C. Phlyctenular conjunctivitis
    D. Lupus vulgaris

121. **Clubbing occurs earliest with**
    A. Mesothelioma of pleura
    B. Fallot's tetralogy
    C. Lung abscess
    D. Bronchiectasis

122. **Commonest sign of aspiration pneumonia is**
    A. Stridor
    B. Tachypnoea
    C. Central cyanosis
    D. Crepitations

123. **All of the following are complicated by cyanosis** *except*
    A. Respiratory failure
    B. Lung abscess
    C. Acute lung injury
    D. Pulmonary thromboembolism

124. **Which is the commonest complication of hyperbaric oxygen therapy**
    A. Pain in the ear
    B. Pneumothorax
    C. Air embolism
    D. Cataracts

Ans: 115-B 116-A 117-A 118-A 119-C 120-D 121-C 122-B 123-B 124-A

125. The dose of which antituberculous drug need not be reduced in severe renal failure
    A. Rifampicin
    B. INH
    C. Pyrazinamide
    D. Streptomycin

126. Emphysema is associated with all *except*
    A. Idiopathic pulmonary haemosiderosis
    B. Pneumoconiosis
    C. Bronchial asthma
    D. Bronchiectasis

127. Risk factor for acquiring tuberculosis is maximum in
    A. Diabetes mellitus
    B. Prolonged corticosteroid therapy
    C. HIV infection
    D. Silicosis

128. Mantoux test may be negative in all *except*
    A. Lymphoma
    B. Corticosteroid therapy
    C. Mumps
    D. Sarcoidosis

129. Bronchial adenoma most commonly present as
    A. Cough
    B. Stridor
    C. Recurrent haemoptysis
    D. Pain chest

130. α-fetoprotein concentration in blood is raised in all *except*
    A. Hepatocellular carcinoma
    B. Glioblastoma multiforme
    C. Foetal anencephaly
    D. Non-seminomatous germ cell tumour of testis

131. Earliest sign of clubbing is
    A. Schamroth's sign
    B. Increased fluctuation at nailbed
    C. Increased pulp tissue
    D. Increase in anteroposterior diameter of nail

132. Nocturnal cough is classically found in all *except*
    A. Post-nasal drip
    B. Tropical eosinophilia
    C. Left ventricular failure
    D. Recurrent laryngeal nerve palsy

133. Bradypnoea is associated with
    A. Narcotic overdose
    B. Acidosis
    C. Pneumonia
    D. Acute lung injury

134. Monophonic rhonchi is classically found in
    A. Chronic bronchitis
    B. Foreign body in bronchus
    C. Emphysema
    D. Bronchial asthma

Ans: 125-A 126-A 127-C 128-C 129-C 130-B 131-B 132-D 133-A 134-B

135. Low-dose aspirin is contraindicated in all *except*

    A. Cerebral haemorrhage   B. Gout

    C. Bronchial asthma   D. Angina pectoris

136. Haemorrhagic pleural effusion is not characteristic of

    A. Systemic lupus erythematosus

    B. Acute pulmonary thromboembolism

    C. Tuberculous effusion

    D. Acute pancreatitis

137. 'Primary' spontaneous pneumothorax is associated with

    A. Tall and thin individuals   B. Non-smokers

    C. Exercise   D. COPD

138. Predominantly left-sided pleural effusion is seen in

    A. Congestive cardiac failure   B. Meig's syndrome

    C. Oesophageal rupture   D. Cirrhosis of liver

139. In allergic asthma, the most important mediator for pathogenesis is

    A. Thromboxane A_2 B. Leukotrienes

    C. Prostaglandins   D. Bradykinin

140. Which of the following antituberculosis drugs should be totally avoided in pregnancy

    A. INH   B. Pyrazinamide

    C. Rifampicin   D. Streptomycin

141. Blood level of theophylline is diminished in associated

    A. Cimetidine therapy   B. Congestive cardiac failure

    C. Smoking   D. Ciprofloxacin therapy

142. Asbestosis may be complicated by all *except*

    A. COPD   B. Mesothelioma of pleura

    C. Bronchogenic carcinoma   D. Pulmonary fibrosis

143. Pulmonary fibrosis is commonly due to complication of

    A. Adriamycin   B. Bleomycin

    C. Vincristine   D. 6-Mercaptopurine

144. Which of the following is correct in type II respiratory failure

    A. $\downarrow Po_2$ and $\downarrow Pco_2$ B. $\downarrow Po_2$ and normal Pco_2

    C. Normal Po_2 and $\uparrow Pco_2$ D. $\downarrow Po_2$ and $\uparrow Pco_2$

Ans: 135-D 136-A 137-A 138-C 139-B 140-D 141-C 142-A 143-B 144-D

145. The commonest cause of acute cor pulmonale is
    A. Lobar consolidation
    B. Pneumothorax
    C. Pulmonary thromboembolism
    D. Fibrosing alveolitis

146. Egg shell calcification in chest X-ray is characteristic of
    A. Tuberculosis   B. Silicosis
    C. Asbestosis   D. Histoplasmosis

147. Exudative pleural effusion is characteristic of
    A. Constrictive pericarditis   B. Nephrotic syndrome
    C. Bronchogenic carcinoma   D. Right ventricular failure

148. Hypercarbia is associated with
    A. Cold-clammy extremities   B. Thready pulse
    C. Intention tremor   D. Systemic hypertension

149. Which of the following drugs is not used in acute asthma
    A. Zafirlukast   B. Terbutaline
    C. Corticosteroids   D. Ipratropium bromide

150. Hypersensitivity pneumonitis is due to
    A. Berylliosis   B. Byssinosis
    C. Asbestosis   D. Bagassosis

151. The next step in a patient of haemoptysis with non-conclusive chest X-ray is
    A. Bronchoscopy   B. HRCT
    C. Bronchography   D. MRI

152. Bronchoalveolar lavage is indicated in evaluation of
    A. Bronchopleural fistula   B. Bronchial asthma
    C. Chronic bronchitis   D. Interstitial lung disease

153. Which variety of lung carcinoma is most commonly associated with hypercalcaemia
    A. Oat cell carcinoma   B. Large cell carcinoma
    C. Squamous cell carcinoma   D. Adenocarcinoma

154. Orthodeoxia is characteristic of
    A. Chronic bronchitis   B. Congestive cardiac failure
    C. Hepatopulmonary syndrome   D. Huge ascites

Ans: 145-C 146-B 147-C 148-D 149-A 150-D 151-B 152-D 153-C 154-C

155. Hepatopulmonary syndrome is characterised by all *except*
    A. Clubbing
    B. P-pulmonale in ECG
    C. Reduction in diffusing capacity of lung
    D. Hypoxia

156. In pleural effusion, an impaired transport of glucose into the pleural space is found in
    A. Myxoedema   B. Tuberculosis
    C. Cirrhosis of liver   D. Rheumatoid arthritis

157. Which of the following is not a recognised ocular complication of sarcoidosis
    A. Scleromalacia perforans   B. Ophthalmoplegia
    C. Uveitis   D. Calcium deposits

158. Which is not manifested as cavitary lung lesion
    A. Wegener's granulomatosis B. Systemic lupus erythematosus
    C. Progressive massive fibrosis D. Tuberculosis

159. Haemoptysis is characteristically seen in all *except*
    A. Goodpasture's syndrome   B. Aspergilloma
    C. Pulmonary vasculitis   D. Byssinosis

160. Cryptogenic fibrosing alveolitis may be associated with all *except*
    A. Chronic constrictive pericarditis
    B. Hashimoto's thyroiditis
    C. Renal tubular acidosis
    D. Chronic active hepatitis

161. Calcification of pleura is not seen in
    A. Tuberculosis   B. Haemothorax
    C. Haemosiderosis   D. Asbestosis

162. Which of the following is not a recognised feature of fibrosing alveolitis
    A. Clubbing   B. Velcro crepitations
    C. Recurrent haemoptysis D. Circulating rheumatoid factor

163. Characteristic feature of pulmonary hypertension does not include
    A. Prominent a-wave in jugular venous pulse
    B. Left parasternal heave
    C. Diastolic shock
    D. Wide splitting of S_2 with loud P_2

Ans: 155-B 156-D 157-A 158-B 159-D 160-A 161-C 162-C 163-D

164. **Acute pulmonary oedema may develop after consumption of all *except***
    A. Procarbazine
    B. Interleukin 2
    C. Methadone
    D. Propoxyphene

165. **Stridor is not a manifestation of**
    A. Tetany
    B. Diphtheria
    C. Foreign body impacted in left main bronchus
    D. Infection by *Haemophilus influenzae*

166. **All of the following commonly affect the upper zone of lung in chest X-ray *except***
    A. Progressive systemic sclerosis
    B. Silicosis
    C. Ankylosing spondylitis
    D. Pulmonary tuberculosis

167. **Haemoptysis following acute pleuritic chest pain and dyspnoea is characteristic of**
    A. Bronchogenic carcinoma
    B. Pulmonary thromboembolism
    C. Pulmonary tuberculosis
    D. Arteriovenous malformations

168. **Scar carcinoma of lung is**
    A. Squamous cell carcinoma
    B. Oat cell carcinoma
    C. Large cell carcinoma
    D. Adenocarcinoma

169. **Hysterical hyperventilation may be mainfested by all *except***
    A. Circumoral numbness
    B. Loss of ankle jerk
    C. Respiratory alkalosis
    D. Chest wall tightness

170. **Ferrugenous bodies are classically seen in**
    A. Berylliosis
    B. Silicosis
    C. Baritosis
    D. Asbestosis

171. **Characteristic body in sarcoidosis is**
    A. Russel bodies
    B. Asteroid bodies
    C. Councilman bodies
    D. Schaumann bodies

172. **Which of the following can be used as Bosentan (endothelin antagonist) analogue in pulmonary hypertension**
    A. Terazosin
    B. Sildenafil
    C. Prostglandin E_1
    D. Donazepril

Ans: 164-A 165-C 166-A 167-B 168-D 169-B 170-D 171-D 172-B

173. **Diffuse alveolar haemorrhage may be an immune reaction to all undermentioned drugs** *except*
    A. Telmisartan
    B. All-trans-retinoic acid
    C. Leukotriene antagonist
    D. Diphenylhydantoin

174. **Which of the following is not responsible for development of interstitial lung disease**
    A. Carbamazepine
    B. Methotrexate
    C. Amiodarone
    D. Carbimazole

175. **Bilateral hilar lymphadenopathy, ankle arthritis and erythema nodosum in sarcoidosis is known as**
    A. Caplan syndrome
    B. Sneddon's syndrome
    C. Leriche's syndrome
    D. Lofgren's syndrome

176. **The most common organism causing pneumonia during mechanical ventilation in the first 4 days of hospitalization is**
    A. *Staphylococcus aureus*
    B. *Streptococcus pneumoniae*
    C. Gram-negative bacilli
    D. *Haemophilus influenzae*

177. **Exposure to rodents may be associated with pneumonia caused by**
    A. *Histoplasma*
    B. *Mycobacterium tuberculosis*
    C. Hantavirus
    D. *Coxiella burnetii*

178. **Which of the following is false in restrictive lung disease**
    A. Decreased vital capacity
    B. Increased residual volume
    C. Decreased functional residual capacity
    D. Decreased total lung capacity

Ans: 173-A 174-D 175-D 176-A 177-C 178-B

5

Neurology

1. Which of the following is not included within 'motor functions'
   A. Nutrition of muscles
   B. Tone and power
   C. Stereognosis
   D. Involuntary movements

2. Which is not a symptom of raised intracranial tension
   A. Altered consciousness
   B. Headache
   C. Non-projectile vomiting
   D. Convulsions

3. Reversible ischaemic neurological deficit (RIND) usually recovers within
   A. 24 hours
   B. 96 hours
   C. 2 weeks
   D. 3 weeks

4. Weber's syndrome is crossed hemiplegia with involvement of
   A. Facial nerve
   B. Oculomotor nerve
   C. Abducent nerve
   D. Vagus nerve

5. In the setting of puerperium, which of the following is most common in producing neurodeficit
   A. Venous sinus thrombosis
   B. Accelerated atherosclerosis
   C. Cerebral embolism
   D. Puerperal sepsis

6. Which of the following is not a feature of 'stage of neural shock' in hemiplegia
   A. Retention of urine
   B. Coma
   C. Absent deep jerks
   D. Hypertonia

7. Neck rigidity is not found in
   A. After epileptic seizure
   B. Meningism
   C. Hysteria
   D. Tetanus

8. Crossed hemiplegia indicates the site of lesion in
   A. Internal capsule
   B. Cortex
   C. Cervical spine
   D. Brainstem

Ans: 1-C 2-C 3-B 4-B 5-A 6-D 7-A 8-D

9. **Which of the following is not a feature of UMN palsy**
   A. Spasticity
   B. Babinski's sign
   C. Clonus
   D. Fasciculations

10. **Neck rigidity may be absent in the presence of**
    A. Hypocalcaemia
    B. Hyperkalaemia
    C. Deep coma
    D. Hyperpyrexia

11. **Which of the following is not a test for cortical sensory function**
    A. Perceptual rivalry
    B. Graphaesthesia
    C. Vibration sensation
    D. Two point localisation

12. **In monoplegia, usually the site of lesion lies in**
    A. Pons
    B. Internal capsule
    C. Cortex
    D. Midbrain

13. **Lasegue's sign is present in**
    A. Cervical spondylosis
    B. Prolapsed intervertebral disc
    C. Duchenne myopathy
    D. Guillain-Barre syndrome

14. **Commonest cerebrovascular accident (CVA) is**
    A. Cerebral haemorrhage
    B. Cerebral thrombosis
    C. Cerebral embolism
    D. Subarachnoid haemorrhage

15. **All are features of pontine haemorrhage** *except*
    A. Disconjugate gaze
    B. Pin-point pupil
    C. Hypothermia
    D. Paralysis

16. **All of the following are sources of cerebral embolism** *except*
    A. Tricuspid incompetence with occasional ectopics
    B. Left ventricular aneurysm
    C. Left atrial myxoma
    D. Subacute bacterial endocarditis

17. **All of the following produce meningism** *except*
    A. Weil's disease
    B. Cerebral malaria
    C. Atypical pneumonia
    D. Enteric fever

18. **All of the following may produce syncope** *except*
    A. Cardiac tamponade
    B. Tight aortic stenosis
    C. Stokes-Adams syndrome
    D. Arrhythmia

Ans: 9-D 10-C 11-C 12-C 13-B 14-B 15-C 16-A 17-B 18-A

19. **Regarding acute transverse myelitis, which is false**
    A. Viral or post-vaccinal
    B. Bladder involvement is very late
    C. Definite upper level of sensory loss
    D. Absence of root pain

20. **Which is not included under 'craniovertebral anomaly'**
    A. Dolicocephaly   B. Klippel-Feil anomaly
    C. Atlantoaxial dislocation   D. Platybasia

21. **Abdominal reflex is lost early in**
    A. Multiple sclerosis   B. Motor neuron disease
    C. Parkinsonism   D. Cerebral diplegia

22. **Which of the following does not produce pure motor paraplegia**
    A. Guillain-Barré syndrome   B. Acute transverse myelitis
    C. Amyotrophic lateral sclerosis   D. Lathyrism

23. **'Paraplegia in flexion' may have all of the following** *except*
    A. Increased tone in flexor groups
    B. Mass reflex
    C. Flexor plantar response
    D. Flexor spasm

24. **Hypertonia is a feature of all** *except*
    A. Tetany   B. Athetosis
    C. Myotonia   D. Chorea

25. **Spastic paraplegia is not produced by**
    A. Guillain-Barré syndrome   B. Cord compression
    C. Lathyrism   D. Acute transverse myelitis

26. **Abdominal reflex is usually retained in**
    A. Obesity   B. Mutiparous woman
    C. Hysteria   D. Lax abdominal wall

27. **Cerebral oedema induced by CVA should not be treated by**
    A. IV mannitol   B. Dexamethasone
    C. Oral glycerol   D. IV frusemide

28. **Tropical spastic paraplegia is caused by**
    A. Bacteria   B. Virus
    C. Toxin   D. Autoimmunity

Ans: 19-B 20-A 21-A 22-B 23-C 24-D 25-A 26-C 27-B 28-B

29. All of the following produce 'cord compression' *except*
    A. Patchy arachnoiditis
    B. Spinal epidural abscess
    C. Subacute combined degeneration
    D. Neurofibroma

30. Froin's loculation syndrome does not have
    A. Xanthochromia
    B. Increased CSF pressure
    C. High protein content
    D. Positive Queckenstedt's test

31. Commonest cause of peripheral neuropathy in India is
    A. Diabetes mellitus
    B. Chronic renal failure
    C. Leprosy
    D. After INH therapy

32. Which of the following is false in subacute combined degeneration
    A. Glossitis
    B. Babinski's sign
    C. Ankle clonus
    D. Anaemia

33. Commonest cause of unilateral foot drop is
    A. Motor neuron disease
    B. Common peroneal nerve palsy
    C. Peripheral neuropathy
    D. Peroneal muscular atrophy

34. Albumino-cytological dissociation is not a feature of
    A. Guillain-Barré syndrome
    B. Acoustic neurofibroma
    C. Froin's loculation syndrome
    D. Meningism

35. Which of the following is involved earliest in diphtheritic neuropathy
    A. Loss of accommodation
    B. Polyneuropathy
    C. Paralysis of soft palate
    D. Abducent palsy

36. Management of choice in Guillain-Barré syndrome is
    A. Immunoglobulin
    B. Cyclophospamide
    C. Corticosteroid
    D. Interferon

37. All of the following produce mononeuritis multiplex *except*
    A. Polyarteritis nodosa
    B. Sarcoidosis
    C. Rheumatoid arthritis
    D. Infectious mononucleosis

38. Muscle sense is increased in all *except*
    A. Myositis
    B. Tabes dorsalis
    C. Polyneuropathy
    D. Subacute combined degeneration

Ans: 29-C 30-B 31-C 32-C 33-B 34-D 35-C 36-A 37-D 38-B

39. **Peripheral neuropathy associated with hypertension is found in**
    A. Acute intermittent porphyria
    B. Amyloidosis
    C. TOCP poisoning
    D. Pyridoxine deficiency

40. **Sensory involvement is not found in**
    A. Encephalitis   B. Myelopathy
    C. Neuropathy   D. Myopathy

41. **Xanthochromia is not a feature of**
    A. Froin's loculation syndrome
    B. Old subarachnoid haemorrhage
    C. Recent intracerebral haemorrhage
    D. Deep jaundice

42. **Posterior column lesion will have**
    A. ↑ tone   B. Intact proprioception
    C. Brisk deep reflexes D. Sensory ataxia

43. **Amantadine does not produce**
    A. Fatty liver   B. Ankle oedema
    C. Seizures   D. Livido reticularis

44. **All of the following produce cerebellar degeneration *except***
    A. Bronchogenic carcinoma   B. Myxoedema
    C. Valproic acid   D. Alcohol

45. **Oculogyric crisis is found in all *except***
    A. Petit mal epilepsy   B. Post-encephalitic parkinsonism
    C. Metoclopramide-induced   D. Millard-Gubler syndrome

46. **Romberg's sign is present in**
    A. Cerebellar ataxia   B. Labyrinthine ataxia
    C. Apraxia   D. Sensory ataxia

47. **Which of the following is not a feature of parkinsonism**
    A. Tremor   B. Rigidity
    C. Normal reflexes   D. Hyperkinesia

48. **Titubation is classically seen in**
    A. Drug-induced dyskinesia B. Parkinsonism
    C. Cerebellar disorder   D. Aortic incompetence

Ans: 39-A 40-D 41-C 42-D 43-A 44-C 45-D 46-D 47-D 48-C

49. **Which is not parkinsonian plus syndrome**
    A. Shy-Drager syndrome   B. Huntington's chorea
    C. Punch-drunk syndrome   D. Normal-pressure hydrocephalus

50. **Pyramidal signs may be associated with**
    A. Post-encephalitic parkinsonism
    B. Atherosclerotic parkinsonism
    C. Punch-drunk syndrome
    D. Idiopathic parkinsonism

51. **Characteristics of 'rigidity' are all** *except*
    A. Uniform affection of flexors and extensors
    B. Indicates disorder of extrapyramidal tract
    C. Flexor plantar response
    D. Increased deep reflexes

52. **'On-off phenomenon' is precipitated by**
    A. Selegiline   B. Levodopa
    C. Amantadine   D. Trihexyphenidyl

53. **Intermittent bulbar palsy is seen in**
    A. Snake bite   B. Myasthenia gravis
    C. Rabies   D. Poliomyelitis

54. **Patient of Down's syndrome may be complicated by all** *except*
    A. Duodenal stenosis   B. Early Alzheimer's disease
    C. Polymyositis   D. Patent ductus arteriosus

55. **Pseudobulbar palsy will have all** *except*
    A. Small, spastic tongue   B. Brisk jaw jerk
    C. Sudden onset   D. Babinski's sign

56. **Which of the following does not produce phakomatosis**
    A. Weber-Christian disease   B. Tuberous sclerosis
    C. von Hippel-Lindau syndrome D. Sturge-Weber disease

57. **CNS involvement of SLE includes all** *except*
    A. Chorea   B. Psychosis
    C. Myoclonus   D. Migraine

58. **Which of the following does not produce wasting of small muscles of hands**
    A. Myopathy   B. Rheumatoid arthritis
    C. Cervical rib   D. Carpal tunnel syndrome

Ans: 49-C 50-A 51-D 52-B 53-B 54-C 55-C 56-A 57-C 58-A

59. **Which is not a manifestation of normal-pressure hydrocephalus**

    A. Urinary incontinence   B. Normal intellectual activity
    C. Ataxia   D. Dementia

60. **Wrist drop is commonly seen in neuropathy induced by**

    A. Vincristine   B. Alcohol
    C. Arsenic   D. Lead

61. **Cafe-au-lait spots are found in all *except***

    A. Albright's disease   B. Subacute bacterial endocarditis
    C. Multiple neurofibromatosis   D. Ataxia telangiectasia

62. **Which of the following does not produce pseudobulbar palsy**

    A. Neurosyphilis
    B. Lacunar infarction
    C. Chronic motor neuron disease
    D. Cerebral atrophy

63. **Which of the following is false regarding aetiology of benign intracranial hypertension**

    A. Hypervitaminosis D   B. Addison's disease
    C. Hypoparathyroidism   D. Corticosteroid withdrawal

64. **Commonest cause of aphasia is**

    A. Hysteria   B. Cerebral infarction
    C. Brain tumour   D. Cerebral haemorrhage

65. **Ptosis is absent in**

    A. Botulism   B. Periodic paralysis
    C. Myopathy of Duchenne type   D. Myasthenia gravis

66. **Which is not a 'primitive reflex'**

    A. Anal reflex   B. Grasp reflex
    C. Sucking reflex   D. Snout reflex

67. **Neurological features of thyrotoxicosis do not include**

    A. Hypokalaemic periodic paralysis
    B. Distal muscle weakness
    C. Exaggerated deep reflex
    D. Pseudoclonus

68. **Fine tremor is found in**

    A. Cerebellar disorder   B. Parkinsonism
    C. Alcoholism   D. Wilson's disease

Ans: 59-B 60-D 61-B 62-A 63-A 64-B 65-C 66-A 67-B 68-C

69. **Neurological feature of myxoedema may be**
    - A. Restlessness
    - B. Transverse myelitis
    - C. Hung-up knee jerk
    - D. Poliomyelitis

70. **Which of the following is not associated with pes cavus**
    - A. Friedreich's ataxia
    - B. Syringomyelia
    - C. Neurofibromatosis
    - D. Poliomyelitis

71. **Miosis is found in all *except***
    - A. Myotonic pupil
    - B. Organophosphorus poisoning
    - C. Old age
    - D. Application of pilocarpine drops

72. **Myxoedema coma is not associated with**
    - A. Hypoxia
    - B. Hyponatraemia
    - C. Hypotension
    - D. Hypocapnia

73. **Flapping tremor is not found in**
    - A. Raised intracranial tension
    - B. Hepatocellular failure
    - C. Hypnotic poisoning
    - D. Severe heart failure

74. **Glasgow coma scale assesses all *except***
    - A. Verbal response
    - B. Eye opening
    - C. Autonomic response
    - D. Motor response

75. **Horner's syndrome includes all of the following *except***
    - A. Complete ptosis
    - B. Constricted pupil
    - C. Anhidrosis
    - D. Enophthalmos

76. **Cause of bilateral facial nerve palsy does not include**
    - A. Myopathy
    - B. Sarcoidosis
    - C. Guillain-Barre syndrome
    - D. Leprosy

77. **Pronator sign, lizard tongue and hung-up deep reflex are found in**
    - A. Myoclonus
    - B. Dystonia
    - C. Hemiballismus
    - D. Chorea

78. **Pendular nystagmus is found in**
    - A. Amblyopia
    - B. Cerebellar disorder
    - C. Pontine glioma
    - D. Phenytoin toxicity

79. **Argyll Robertson pupil is found in all *except***
    - A. Wernicke's encephalopathy
    - B. Multiple sclerosis
    - C. Cerebral haemorrhage
    - D. Pinealomas

Ans: 69-C 70-C 71-A 72-D 73-A 74-C 75-A 76-A 77-D 78-A 79-C

80. **Corneal reflex tests the integrity of**

    A. Optic nerve
    C. Trochlear nerve
    B. Facial nerve
    D. Trigeminal nerve

81. **All of the following may produce papilloedema** *except*

    A. Guillain-Barre syndrome
    B. Malignant hypertension
    C. Cavernous sinus thrombosis
    D. Hypoxia

82. **Lesion in athetosis lies in**

    A. Caudate nucleus
    C. Red nucleus
    B. Putamen
    D. Substantia nigra

83. **Commonest cause of abducent nerve palsy is**

    A. Brain tumour
    C. Raised intracranial tension
    B. Diabetes mellitus
    D. Gradenigo's syndrome

84. **Which of the following does not fit in 'Ramsay Hunt syndrome'**

    A. LMN type of VIIth nerve palsy
    B. Loss of taste sensation of anterior 2/3rd of tongue
    C. Diminished auditory acuity
    D. Herpetic rash on tympanic membrane

85. **Optic neuritis may be produced by all** *except*

    A. Ethambutol
    C. Multiple sclerosis
    B. Leprosy
    D. Syphilis

86. **All of the following may develop into chorea** *except*

    A. Hyponatraemia
    C. Wilson's disease
    B. Rheumatic fever
    D. Thyrotoxicosis

87. **Internuclear ophthalmoplegia results from**

    A. III, IV, VIth nerve palsy
    B. Malignant exophthalmos
    C. Lesion in medial longitudinal bundle
    D. Ocular myopathy

88. **Which of the following does not produce fasciculation**

    A. Recovery phase of poliomyelitis
    B. Organophosphorus poisoning
    C. Chronic motor neuron disease
    D. Hereditary spastic paraplegia

Ans: 80-D 81-D 82-B 83-C 84-C 85-B 86-A 87-C 88-D

89. **True hypertrophy of muscles is found in all** *except*
    A. Duchenne type muscular dystrophy
    B. Manual labourers
    C. Myotonia
    D. Athletes

90. **Root value of 'plantar response' is**
    A. L_5 B. $S_{1,2}$
    C. S_1 D. L_5, S_1

91. **Myopathy is best diagnosed by**
    A. Muscle enzyme study   B. Nerve conduction study
    C. Muscle biopsy   D. Electromyography

92. **Trismus is seen in all of the following** *except*
    A. Tetanus
    B. Hydrophidae group of snake bite
    C. Diphtheria
    D. Quinsy

93. **Atrophy in Duchenne myopathy is classically seen in**
    A. Pectoralis major   B. Deltoid
    C. Infraspinatus   D. Calf muscles

94. **Limb-girdle type myopathy inherits the disease as**
    A. X-linked dominant   B. Autosomal recessive
    C. X-linked recessive   D. Autosomal dominant

95. **Delayed relaxation of ankle jerk is seen in all** *except*
    A. Parkinsonism   B. Gross pedal oedema
    C. Myxoedema   D. Tabes dorsalis

96. **Main d' accoucheur is seen in**
    A. Hypocalcaemia   B. Hyperkalaemia
    C. Hyponatraemia   D. Hypercalcaemia

97. **Proximal muscle weakness is not produced by**
    A. Guillain-Barre syndrome   B. Leprosy
    C. Diabetic amyotrophy   D. Polymyositis

98. **Myotonia dystrophica has all of the following morphological features** *except*
    A. Frontal baldness   B. Ptosis
    C. Testicular atroply   D. Brachycephaly

Ans: 89-A 90-C 91-C 92-C 93-A 94-B 95-D 96-A 97-B 98-D

99. **Inversion of supinator jerk indicates the lesion at**
    A. $C_{3,4}$ B. $C_{4,5}$
    C. $C_{5,6}$ D. $C_{6,7}$

100. **Waddling gait is seen in all *except***
    A. Advanced pregnancy
    B. Charcot-Marie-Tooth disease
    C. Duchenne muscular dystrophy
    D. Huge ascites

101. **Vibration sensation is lost early in**
    A. Leprosy   B. Alcoholic polyneuropathy
    C. Diabetes mellitus   D. Multiple sclerosis

102. **Most common psychological disorder in myxoedema is**
    A. Phobia   B. Paranoia
    C. Mania   D. Depression

103. **Presence of Babinski's sign with loss of ankle jerk is found in all *except***
    A. Friedreich's ataxia   B. Subacute combined degeneration
    C. Hepatic precoma   D. Taboparesis

104. **Which is abnormal regarding normal CSF findings**
    A. Protein content 20–40 mg%
    B. Sugar content 40–80 mg%
    C. Pressure 60–150 mm of CSF in sitting position
    D. Chloride content 720–750 mg%

105. **Atypical feature of Guillain-Barré syndrome is**
    A. SIADH   B. Optic neuritis
    C. Pseudobulbar palsy   D. Convulsions

106. **The site of lesion in Korsakoff's psychosis is**
    A. Corpus striatum   B. Mammillary bodies
    C. Frontal lobe   D. Temporal lobe

107. **Babinski's sign is not found in**
    A. Electroconvulsive therapy   B. Peripheral neuropathy
    C. Hypoglycaemic coma   D. Marathon runner

108. **Korsakoff's psychosis does not have the feature like**
    A. Retrograde amnesia   B. Defect in learning
    C. Loss of immediate recall   D. Confabulation

Ans: 99-C 100-B 101-C 102-D 103-C 104-C 105-A 106-B 107-B 108-C

109. Perforating ulcer in sole of foot is found in all *except*

    A. Diabetic neuropathy   B. Tabes dorsalis

    C. Leprosy   D. Raynaud's disease

110. Which of the following remains normal in leprosy

    A. EMG   B. Sensory functions

    C. Cerebellar functions   D. Proprioception

111. In cerebral malaria, which of the following should not be given

    A. IV mannitol   B. Glucocorticoids

    C. 5% dextrose   D. IV quinine

112. Berry aneurysm may be associated with all *except*

    A. Polycystic kidney   B. Coarctation of aorta

    C. Ehlers-Danlos syndrome   D. Takayasu's disease

113. Congenital abnormality produced by lithium therapy is

    A. Anencephaly   B. Heart valve abnormalities

    C. Mental retardation   D. Limb shortening

114. Drug of choice in obsessive-compulsive psychosis is

    A. Carbamazepine   B. Haloperidol

    C. Lithium   D. Clomipramine

115. Which does not produce hypoglycorrhachia (low CSF sugar)

    A. Pyogenic meningitis   B. Tuberculous meningitis

    C. Hypoglycaemia   D. Viral meningitis

116. The drug most beneficial in enuresis of a 10-year-old boy is

    A. Chlorpromazine   B. Trimipramine

    C. Benzodiazepines   D. Haloperidol

117. Neuroleptic malignant syndrome has all the following features *except*

    A. Autonomic dysfunction

    B. Pseudoparkinsonism

    C. Hyperpyrexia

    D. Haloperidol is the mainstay of treatment

118. All of the following are recognised lithium toxicity *except*

    A. Nephrogenic diabetes insipidus

    B. Hypothyroidism

    C. Ataxia

    D. Thrombocytopenia

Ans: 109-D 110-C 111-B 112-D 113-B 114-D 115-D 116-B 117-D 118-D

119. 'India ink preparation' in CSF helps in the diagnosis of

A. Lymphocytic choriomeningitis
B. Herpes simplex virus meningitis
C. Cryptococcal meningitis
D. Coxsackie virus meningitis

120. Maligant hyperthermia may be produced by all *except*

A. Dantrolene
B. Methoxyflurane
C. Succinylcholine
D. Halothane

121. Lymphocytic pleocytosis in CSF is not found in

A. Meningococcal meningitis
B. Neurosarcoidosis
C. Multiple sclerosis
D. Viral meningitis

122. All of the following are seen in bulimia *except*

A. Caries teeth
B. Amenorrhoea
C. Emaciation
D. Elevated serum amylase

123. Lithium is not used in

A. Polycythaemia vera
B. Mania
C. SIADH
D. Cluster headache

124. Narcolepsy is not associated with

A. Sleep paralysis
B. Epilepsy
C. Hypnagogic hallucination
D. Cataplexy

125. Which of the following is false in Gerstmann's syndrome

A. Agraphia
B. Lesion in dominant parietal lobe
C. Aphasia
D. Acalculia

126. Prophylaxis of migraine may be done by

A. Atenolol
B. Phenytoin
C. Verapamil
D. Sumatriptan

127. Reversible cause of dementia is

A. Post-encephalitic
B. Multi-infarct dementia
C. Huntington's chorea
D. Alzheimer's disease

128. Which of the following is false in cluster headache

A. Male dominance
B. Propranolol is effective in prophylaxis
C. Absence of hereditary predisposition
D. Periorbital pain

Ans: 119-C 120-A 121-A 122-C 123-A 124-B 125-C 126-C 127-A 128-B

129. **Palatal myoclonus is seen in**
    A. Multiple sclerosis   B. Epilepsy
    C. Eaton-Lambert syndrome   D. Cerebellar infarction

130. **Which of the following is false regarding migraine**
    A. Hereditary predisposition
    B. Common migraine has aura
    C. Common in women
    D. Hemicranial headache

131. **Hypersomnolence is found in all *except***
    A. Subdular haematoma   B. Encephalitis lethargica
    C. Trypanosomiasis   D. Pickwickian syndrome

132. **'Hippus' is**
    A. Unequal pupil
    B. Synonymous with pin-point pupil
    C. Abnormal neurological movement disorder
    D. Spontaneous phasic constriction and dilatation of pupil

133. **Apneustic breathing is seen in lesion of**
    A. Midbrain   B. Upper pons
    C. Lower pons   D. Medulla

134. **Jaw claudication is not characteristic of**
    A. Temporomandibular joint dysfunction
    B. Trigeminal neuralgia
    C. Giant cell arteritis
    D. Glossopharyngeal neuralgia

135. **Xanthopsia is found in**
    A. Aura phase of migraine   B. Lesion in visual cortex
    C. Digitalis toxicity   D. Cerebellar infarction

136. **Meralgia paraesthetica is characterised by all *except***
    A. A peculiar numb, tingling sensation in upper lateral thigh
    B. May occur spontaneously
    C. Seen in tall, slender persons
    D. Quite often remits spontaneously

137. **The most consistent early physical sign evoked in a cerebello-pontine angle tumour is**
    A. Loss of corneal reflex   B. Cerebellar signs
    C. Facial nerve palsy   D. Pyramidal signs

Ans: 129-D 130-B 131-A 132-D 133-C 134-D 135-C 136-C 137-A

138. The most common lacunar syndrome in clinical practice is
    A. Dysarthria-clumsy hand syndrome
    B. Pure motor hemiparesis
    C. Pure sensory stroke
    D. Ataxic-hemiparesis

139. Which is not characteristic of lateral medullary syndrome (Wallenberg's syndrome)
    A. Horner's syndrome   B. Hiccough
    C. Pyramidal lesion   D. Ataxia

140. In trochlear nerve palsy, the patient complains of diplopia while
    A. Reading a book
    B. Looking in front
    C. Looking to the roof
    D. Looking sideways by the affected eye

141. Lhermitte's sign is not found in
    A. Cervical spondylosis   B. Syringomyelia
    C. Motor neuron disease   D. Multiple sclerosis

142. MRI is preferred over CT scan of brain in all *except*
    A. Posterior fossa tumours   B. Multiple sclerosis
    C. Pituitary tumours   D. Clacification within a lesion

143. Oculomotor nerve palsy with spared pupil is classically seen in
    A. Tuberculous meningitis   B. Diabetes mellitus
    C. Multiple sclerosis   D. Brain tumour

144. Transient ischaemic attack (TIA) stamps the process as
    A. Embolic   B. Demyelinating
    C. Haemorrhagic   D. Inflammatory

145. Commonest intracranial tumour in children is
    A. Medulloblastoma   B. Meningioma
    C. Metastatic carcinoma   D. Cerebellar haemangioblastoma

146. Slow virus CNS infections are all *except*
    A. Progressive multifocal leukoencephalopathy
    B. Subacute sclerosing panencephalitis (SSPE)
    C. Leukodystrophy
    D. Tropical spastic paraplegia

Ans: 138-B 139-C 140-A 141-C 142-D 143-B 144-A 145-A 146-C

147. **The earliest skin lesion in tuberous sclerosis is**
    A. White spots over trunk and limbs
    B. Adenoma sebaceum
    C. Pompholyx
    D. Shagreen patch

148. **All are true regarding Alzheimer's disease** *except*
    A. Microscopically 'neurofibrillary tangles' are found
    B. Donazepril is used in treatment
    C. Aluminium silicate is found in neuritic plaques
    D. Biochemically cortical 'choline acetyltransferase' is increased

149. **Nimodipine used in subarachnoid haemorrhage**
    A. Prevents excruciating nuchal headache
    B. Prevents vasospasm
    C. Hastens absorption of blood from CSF
    D. Prevents rebleeding

150. **Regarding subacute sclerosing panencephalitis (SSPE), all are true** *except*
    A. Isoprinosine is the drug of choice
    B. Affects at 5–15 yrs age
    C. CSF anti-mumps antibody level is high
    D. MRI shows multifocal white matter lesion

151. **'Candle gutterings' on the walls of the ventricles are seen in CT scan in**
    A. Alzheimer's disease   B. Tuberous sclerosis
    C. Leucodystrophy   D. Cerebral palsy

152. **Which of the following is not included in the triad of tuberous sclerosis**
    A. Phakomatosis   B. Mental retardation
    C. Adenoma sebaceum   D. Seizures

153. **The common sites of meningioma are all** *except*
    A. Sylvian fissure   B. Olfactory groove
    C. Cerebello-pontine angle   D. Over visual cortex

154. **Which is not a PRION disease**
    A. Gerstmann-Straussler-Scheinker syndrome
    B. Rubella panencephalitis
    C. Creutzfeldt-Jakob disease
    D. Kuru

Ans: 147-A 148-D 149-B 150-C 151-B 152-A 153-D 154-B

155. Which organism commonly produces meningitis in an adolescent
    A. *E. coli*
    B. *Pneumococcus*
    C. *Meningococcous*
    D. *H. influenzae*

156. ' Railroad track' calcification in X-ray skull is found in
    A. von Recklinghausen's disease
    B. Ataxia telangiectasia
    C. Sturge-Weber disease
    D. Tuberous sclerosis

157. α-bungarotoxin is associated with neuroparalysis in
    A. Elapidae group snake bite
    B. Bolulinus poisoning
    C. Periodic paralysis
    D. Lathyrism

158. Which of the following does not produce thickened peripheral nerves
    A. Chronic Guillain-Barre syndrome
    B. Refsum's disease
    C. Leprosy
    D. Alcoholic polyneuropathy

159. Selective serotonin reuptake inhibitors (SSRI) are all *except*
    A. Paroxetine
    B. Fluvoxamine
    C. Sertraline
    D. Fluoxetine

160. Brushfield's spots in iris are seen in
    A. Noonan's syndrome
    B. Down's syndrome
    C. Turner's syndrome
    D. Klinefelter's syndrome

161. Therapeutic range of phenytoin is
    A. 5–10 μg/ml
    B. 10–20 μg/ml
    C. 20–30 μg/ml
    D. 30–40 μg/ml

162. Tensilon test improves the muscle weakness in
    A. Motor neuron disease
    B. Myopathy
    C. Myasthenia gravis
    D. Polymyositis

163. All of the following are antiepileptic drugs *except*
    A. Lubeluzole
    B. Lamotrigine
    C. Felbamate
    D. Vigabatrin

164. Regarding dermatomyositis, which one is false
    A. Lilac-coloured knee and elbow is known as Gottron's sign
    B. Heliotrope rash over face is characteristic
    C. May be associated with malignancy
    D. Childhood disease is associated with vascular damage

Ans: 155-C 156-C 157-A 158-D 159-C 160-B 161-B 162-C 163-A 164-A

165. The commonest cause of convulsion in a child (2–12 yrs) is
- A. Encephalitis
- B. Trauma
- C. Epilepsy
- D. Febrile

166. Refsum's disease is associated with all *except*
- A. Tissue accumulation of phytanic acid
- B. Deafness
- C. Acanthocytosis of RBC
- D. Retinitis pigmentosa

167. All of the following may develop into endocrine myopathy *except*
- A. Hypothyroidism
- B. Cushing's syndrome
- C. Hyperthyroidism
- D. Diabetes mellitus

168. Increased jaw jerk is seen in
- A. Syringomyelia
- B. Bulbar palsy
- C. Hyperthyroidism
- D. Chronic motor neuron disease

169. Uncinate fits are characteristically seen in tumour of
- A. Occipital lobe
- B. Temporal lobe
- C. Parietal lobe
- D. Frontal lobe

170. Migraine is not associated with
- A. Dysphasia
- B. Diplopia
- C. Seizures
- D. Paraesthesia

171. Which of the following is not a feature of syringobulbia
- A. Spastic tongue
- B. Dysphagia
- C. Nasal regurgitation
- D. Dysarthria

172. EEG findings showing slow waves, spikes and 'burst suppression' are characteristic of
- A. Infantile spasm
- B. Absence seizures
- C. Tonic seizures
- D. Myoclonic seizures

173. Hiccough occurs in all of the following *except*
- A. Wallenberg's syndrome
- B. Acute renal failure
- C. Oesophagitis
- D. Diaphragmatic pleurisy

Ans: 165-C 166-C 167-D 168-D 169-B 170-C 171-A 172-A 173-C

174. **Which of the following is false regarding Eaton-Lambert syndrome**
    A. Repeated efforts increase muscle strength
    B. Deep reflexes are depressed
    C. Guanidine hydrochloride is the treatment of choice
    D. Ocular muscles are commonly involved

175. **Tabes dorsalis presents with all** *except*
    A. Waddling gait   B. Argyll Robertson pupil
    C. Loss of ankle jerk   D. Sensory dysfunction

176. **Multiple sclerosis is not associated with**
    A. Temporal pallor of optic disc B. Papilloedema
    C. Nystagmus   D. Aphasia

177. **'Organic brain syndrome' may be produced by**
    A. Macrolides   B. Aminoglycosides
    C. Cephalosporins   D. Quinolones

178. **Oppenheim's gait is characteristic of**
    A. Peripheral neuropathy   B. Duchenne myopathy
    C. Multiple sclerosis   D. Hysteria

179. **Carbamazepine is used in all of the following** *except*
    A. Post-herpetic neuralgia B. Alcohol withdrawal
    C. Mania   D. Schizophrenia

180. **Neurofibromatosis leads to an increased risk of having all of the following** *except*
    A. Phaeochromocytoma   B. Meningioma
    C. Acoustic neuroma   D. Ependymoma

181. **Which of the following is not a part of Miller-Fisher syndrome**
    A. Ataxia   B. Apraxia
    C. Areflexia   D. External ophthalmoplegia

182. **Which of the following produces wrist drop**
    A. Poliomyelitis   B. Carpal tunnel syndrome
    C. Syringomyelia   D. Radial nerve palsy

183. **Bromocriptine is not useful in the treatment of**
    A. Alzheimer's disease   B. Acromegaly
    C. Parkinsonism   D. Infertility

Ans: 174-D 175-A 176-B 177-D 178-C 179-B 180-D 181-B 182-D   183-A

184. In health, intracranial calcification may be seen in all *except*

A. Pineal body
B. Choroid plexus
C. Basal ganglia
D. Dura mater

185. Down-beating nystagmus is seen in

A. Vestibular lesion
B. Labyrinthine lesion
C. Midbrain lesion
D. Posterior fossa lesion

186. The commonest type of neurofibroma is associated with

A. Scoliosis
B. Meningioma
C. Optic glioma
D. Acoustic neuroma

187. Familial periodic paralysis may be seen in all *except*

A. Normokalaemia
B. Hyperkalaemia
C. Hypercalcaemia
D. Hypokalaemia

188. Which of the following does not produce wasting of small muscles of hands

A. Duchenue muscular dystrophy
B. Thoracic inlet syndrome
C. Rheumatoid arthritis
D. Amyotrophic lateral sclerosis

189. Acoustic neuroma most likely leads to paralysis of

A. IVth cranial nerve
B. VIth cranial nerve
C. VIIth cranial nerve
D. Xth cranial nerve

190. Disorder of language of cerebral origin is

A. Dysarthria
B. Dysphonia
C. Aphasia
D. Monotonous speech

191. 3-Hz spike-and-wave discharge in EEG during the seizure is diagnostic of

A. Generalised tonic clonic
B. Petit mal
C. Infantile spasm
D. Complex partial

192. Characteristic of LMN lesion is

A. Weakness and spasticity
B. Absent superficial reflex
C. Equivocal plantar response
D. Brisk deep reflexes

193. Which of the following is not an antiplatelet drug

A. Ticlopidine
B. Pentoxifylline
C. Clopidogrel
D. Aspirin

Ans: 184-C 185-D 186-A 187-C 188-A 189-C 190-C 191-B 192-B 193-B

194. **Commonest cause of subarachnoid haemorrhage is**
    A. Rupture of arteriovenous malformations
    B. Systemic hypertension
    C. Emotional excitement
    D. Berry aneurysm rupture

195. **Chromosomal anomaly associated with Alzheimer's disease is**
    A. Trisomy-13   B. Trisomy-18
    C. Trisomy-21   D. Turner's syndrome

196. **Ptosis with dialated pupil is observed in**
    A. Horner's syndrome   B. Myasthenia gravis
    C. Oculomotor palsy   D. Botulism

197. **Todd's palsy is characteristic of**
    A. Transient ischaemic attack
    B. Epilepsy
    C. Subarachnoid haemorrhage
    D. Head injury

198. **Commonest cause of anisocoria is**
    A. Oculomotor palsy
    B. Application of mydriatic to one eye
    C. Horner's syndrome
    D. Huchinson's pupil

199. **Internuclear ophthalmoplegia is commonly due to**
    A. Multiple sclerosis   B. Ocular myopathy
    C. Myasthenia grvis   D. Diabetes mellitus

200. **The most common site of hypertensive intracranial bleeding is**
    A. Putamen   B. Midbrain
    C. Cerebellum   D. Thalamus

201. **Drug-induced myopathy may result from all** *except*
    A. Zidovudine   B. Emetine
    C. Febuxostat   D. Lovastatin

202. **Dilator pupillae is supplied by**
    A. Optic nerve
    B. Cholinergic fibres of oculomotor nerve
    C. Trochlear nerve
    D. Adrenergic fibres of oculomotor nerve

Ans: 194-D 195-C 196-C 197-B 198-B 199-A 200-A 201-C 202-D

203. Brain biopsy in rabies demonstrates
- A. Lewy bodies
- B. Negri bodies
- C. Schaumann bodies
- D. Asteroid bodies

204. In lathyrism, the toxin responsible for development of neuroparalysis is
- A. Beta oxalyl amino alanine
- B. Aflatoxin
- C. Pyrrolizidine alkaloids
- D. Thiocyanates

205. Complication of phenytoin does not include
- A. Ataxia
- B. Osteomalacia
- C. Megaloblastic anaemia
- D. Hyperglycaemia

206. All are the complications of oral contraceptive pills *except*
- A. Venous thrombosis
- B. Cerebral haemorrhage
- C. Cerebral infarction
- D. Acute myocardial infarction

207. All of the following may cause peripheral neuropathy *except*
- A. Nitrofurantoin
- B. Vincristine
- C. Methotrexate
- D. INH

208. Which of the following may develop into paranoid psychosis
- A. Carbamazepine
- B. Cocaine
- C. Amphetamines
- D. Flumazenil

209. Right middle cerebral artery territory infarction usually does not feature
- A. Coma
- B. Aphasia
- C. Facial weakness
- D. Hemiparesis

210. Sarcoidosis commonly involves the cranial nerve
- A. IIIrd
- B. Vth
- C. VIIth
- D. Xth

211. Significant loss of vision in a hypertensive patient may be due to all *except*
- A. Papilloedema
- B. Retinal haemorrhage
- C. Infarction of occipital lobe
- D. Ischaemic optic neuropathy

212. Ptosis associated with diplopia and diminished movement of eyeball is due to
- A. Myasthenia gravis
- B. Periodic paralysis
- C. Elapidae snake bite
- D. Oculomotor palsy

Ans: 203-B 204-A 205-D 206-B 207-C 208-C 209-B 210-C 211-A 212-D

213. **Bromocriptine is used in all of the following *except***
    A. Galactorrhoea
    B. Acromegaly
    C. Gynaecomastia
    D. Parkinsonism

214. **Horner's syndrome manifests as**
    A. Complete ptosis + miosis
    B. Partial ptosis + miosis
    C. Anhidrosis + mydriasis
    D. Hydrosis + miosis

215. **CSF is absorbed by arachnoid villi which are mainly present in**
    A. Superior sagittal sinus
    B. Fourth ventricle
    C. Transverse sinus
    D. Inferior sagittal sinus

216. **Chronic fatigue syndrome is fundamentally a**
    A. Neuroendocrine disorder
    B. Immune disorder
    C. Psychiatric disorder
    D. Metabolic disorder

217. **Heerfordt's syndrome is uveoparotid fever with cranial nerve palsy, and is seen in**
    A. Leprosy
    B. Tuberculosis
    C. Mikulicz's syndrome
    D. Sarcoidosis

218. **Which group of muscles are almost never affected in polymyositis**
    A. Ocular muscles
    B. Proximal limb muscles
    C. Anterior neck muscles
    D. Pharyngeal muscles

219. **Commonest presentation of neurocysticercosis is**
    A. Focal neurodeficit
    B. Blindness
    C. Radioculomyelopathy
    D. Convulsions

220. **"Bull's-eye maculopathy" is characteristic toxicity of**
    A. Ethambutol
    B. Amiodarone
    C. Chloroquine
    D. Probenecid

221. **Thrombosis of left middle cerebral artery may give rise to**
    A. Diplopia
    B. Paralysis of conjugate gaze towards left
    C. Right homonymous hemianopia
    D. Hemiplegia of the right side where affection of leg is more than arm

Ans: 213-C 214-B 215-A 216-C 217-D 218-A 219-D 220-C 221-C

222. Chorea may develop from consumption of
  A. Reserpine
  B. Oral contraceptive pills
  C. Pindolol
  D. Ursodeoxycolic acid

223. Anterior horn cell disease is
  A. Myasthenia gravis
  B. Progressive muscular atrophy
  C. Tabes dorsalis
  D. Botulism

224. Phenytoin toxicity may result in all *except*
  A. Pendular nystagmus
  B. Cerebellar syndrome
  C. Pseudolymphoma
  D. Megaloblastic anaemia

225. Which of the following is false in polymyositis
  A. Has a good prognosis in children
  B. Myoglobinuria may be associated with
  C. Wasting of small muscles of the hand is characteristic
  D. A component of mixed connective tissue disease

226. Charcot (neuropathic) joint is a recognised complication of all *except*,
  A. Diabetes mellitus
  B. Tabes dorsalis
  C. Syringomyelia
  D. Friedreich's ataxia

227. Unilateral ptosis is characteristic of all *except*
  A. Cavernous sinus thrombosis
  B. Cluster headache
  C. Bell's palsy
  D. Syringobulbia

228. Pseudobulbar palsy is not associated with
  A. Emotional incontinence
  B. Extensor plantar response
  C. Flaccid dysarthria
  D. Masked facies

229. Dermatoglyphics with obtuse ATD angle is characteristic of
  A. Turner's syndrome
  B. Down's syndrome
  C. Klinefelter's syndrome
  D. Noonan's syndrome

230. Alcohol withdrawal is not associated with
  A. Confabulation
  B. Tremor
  C. Visual hallucinations
  D. Perspiration

231. In schizophrenia, a better prognosis is indicated by
  A. Depression
  B. Early onset
  C. Visual hallucinations
  D. Passivity feelings

Ans: 222-B 223-B 224-A 225-C 226-D 227-C 228-C 229-B 230-A 231-A

232. **Which is not true in Korsakoff's syndrome**
   - A. Loss of recent memory
   - B. Associated with lacunar infarction
   - C. Confabulation
   - D. Presence of nystagmus

233. **Carotid artery stenosis gives rise to**
   - A. Ipsilateral hemiplegia
   - B. Drop attacks
   - C. Diplopia
   - D. Transient ipsilateral monocular blindness

234. **Muscle pain is not characteristic of**
   - A. McArdle's disease (muscle phosphorylase deficiency)
   - B. Guillain-Barre syndrome
   - C. Steroid myopathy
   - D. Amyotrophic lateral sclerosis

235. **All are recognised side effects of lithium** *except*
   - A. Diarrhoea
   - B. Hypothyroidism
   - C. Ataxia
   - D. Onycholysis

236. **Astasia-abasia is known as**
   - A. Hysterical gait disorder
   - B. Muscle contraction in myotonia
   - C. Asthenia in motor neuron disease
   - D. Dementia in AIDS

237. **Gilles de la Tourette syndrome encompasses all** *except*
   - A. Multiple tics
   - B. Coprolalia
   - C. Dementia
   - D. Relief by haloperidol

238. **Ocular bobbing is often diagnostic of bilateral damage of**
   - A. Cerebral cortex
   - B. Midbrain
   - C. Internal capsule
   - D. Pons

239. **Dementia pugilistica develops as a result of**
   - A. 'Normal-pressure' hydrocephalus
   - B. Head trauma in professional boxers
   - C. Alzheimer's disease
   - D. Huntington's disease

240. **Presence of acanthocytosis of RBC, retinitis pigmentosa and ataxia is suggestive of**
   - A. Abetalipoproteinaemia
   - B. Gaucher's disease
   - C. Mucopolysaccharidoses
   - D. Swiss type agammaglobulinaemia

Ans: 232-B 233-D 234-C 235-D 236-A 237-C 238-D 239-B 240-A

241. Cataract is not characteristic of
    A. Wilson's disease
    B. Haemochromatosis
    C. Myotonic dystrophy
    D. Galactosaemia

242. Internuclear ophthalmoplegia results from damage of
    A. Sympathetic nervous system
    B. Ciliary ganglion
    C. Medial longitudinal fasciculus
    D. Oculomotor nerve

243. Commonest intracranial tumour is
    A. Astrocytoma
    B. Glioblastoma
    C. Meningioma
    D. Metastatic

244. The dermatome at nipple is
    A. C_8
    B. T_7
    C. T_2
    D. T_4

245. 'Locked-in syndrome' occurs in lesion of
    A. Ventral pons
    B. Cortex
    C. Internal capsule
    D. Thalamus

246. Fear of relapse in cancer survivors is known as
    A. Dandy-Walker syndrome
    B. Damocles syndrome
    C. Gillespie's syndrome
    D. Da Costa's syndrome

247. Among the following, which is most common adult muscular dystrophy
    A. Becker muscular dystrophy
    B. Facioscapulohumeral dystrophy
    C. Duchenne muscular dystrophy
    D. Myotonic dystrophy

248. Which of the following is homologue of Hoffman's sign of upper extremity
    A. Chaddock's sign
    B. Gonda sign
    C. Babinski's sign
    D. Rossolimo's sign

249. The lobe of brain primarily affected in herpes simplex encephalitis is
    A. Temporal
    B. Frontal
    C. Parietal
    D. Occipital

Ans: 241-B 242-C 243-D 244-D 245-A 246-B 247-D 248-D 249-A

73. **All are true in severe PS** *except*
    A. The ejection click goes away from S_1
    B. Intensity of murmur is maximum towards S_2
    C. Gap between A_2 and P_2 is increased
    D. A_2 is gradually ro... murmur

74. **Aortic arch syndrome is not associated with**
    A. Diminished pulses in ... extremity
    B. Disturbances in vision
    C. Intermittent claudication
    D. Systemic hypertension

75. ... of the following drugs is not used in hypoxic spells of Fallot's tetralogy
    A. Phenylephrine   B. Amiodarone
    C. Propranolol   D. Morphine

76. **The disease with male preponderance is**
    A. Coarctation of aorta
    B. Primary pulmonary hypertension
    C. ...
    D. ...

77. The ... roentgenogram diagnoses
    A. ...   B. VSD
    C. ...   D. AS

78. **Varying intensity of S_1 is found in all** *except*
    A. ...   B. Ventricular tachycardia
    C. Complete heart block   D. Atrial fibrillation

79. **Double ... hypertrophic cardiomyopathy is mainly due to**
    A. Palpable ...   B. Muscle tremor
    C. ... snap   D. Palpable S_3

80. ... **is found in all** *except*
    A. Digitalis overdose   B. Tachycardia
    C. ...valve calcification   D. Left atrial failure

81. '...' **is not found in**
    A. ...   B. ...
    C. ...   D. VSD

Ans: 73-A 74-C 75-B 76-A 77-C 78-A 79-A 80-B 81-B

35. Which of the following is not true in thrombasthenia
- A. Prolonged bleeding time
- B. Normal platelet count
- C. Platelet aggregation defect
- D. Prolonged clotting time

36. Which of the following is not associated with hypersplenism
- A. Anaemia
- B. Fatty marrow in bone marrow
- C. Pancytopenia
- D. Reversibility by splenectomy

37. Splenectomy is virtually curative in *except*
- A. Hereditary spherocytosis
- B. Idiopathic thrombocytopenic purpura (ITP)
- C. Thalassaemia
- D. Hereditary spherocytosis

38. In chronic granulomatous disease, which is false
- A. Predisposition to infection by staphylococci
- B. Neutrophil count is normal
- C. Immunity to phagocytosis
- D. Diagnosed by amount of nitroblue tetrazolium reduction

39. Thymoma may be associated with all of the following *except*
- A. Cushing's syndrome
- B. Hypergammaglobulinaemia
- C. Myasthenia gravis
- D. Pure red cell aplasia

40. Red cell osmotic fragility is increased in
- A. Thalassaemia major
- B. Hereditary spherocytosis
- C. HbC disease
- D. Iron deficiency anaemia

41. Plummer-Vinson syndrome is not associated with
- A. Angular stomatitis
- B. Splenomegaly
- C. Glossitis
- D. Post-cricoid web

42. Warm-antibody mediated haemolysis is not found in
- A. SLE
- B. Infectious mononucleosis
- C. Non-Hodgkin's lymphoma
- D. Chronic lymphatic leukaemia

43. Haemolytic anaemia is not produced by diseases *except*
- A. Penicillin
- B. Lithium
- C. Quinidine
- D. Methyldopa

Ans: 35-D 36-B 37-D 38-C 39-B 40-B 41-C 42-D 43-B

6 Nephrology

44. All of the following are true in paroxysmal nocturnal haemoglobinuria (PNH) except
A. Low leucocyte alkaline phosphatase
B. Elevated LDH
C. Positive acidified serum lysis (HAM) test

45. Sideroblastic anaemia may be treated by all except
A. Pyridoxine B. Hydroxyurea
C. Pyraemia

46. Which of the following is not true in paroxysmal cold haemoglobinuria
A. Associated with mycoplasma infection
B. IgG antibody mediated
C. Precipitated by exposure to cold

47. Myelophthisic anaemia is characterised by all except
A. Leucoerythroblastic blood picture

1. Streptococcal pyoderma may be associated with all except
A. Pyaemia B. Acute rheumatic fever
C. Mild fever D. Acute glomerulonephritis (AGN)

2. All are recognised causes of chronic renal failure (CRF) except
A. Snake bite B. Malignant hypertension
C. Diabetes mellitus D. Obstructive uropathy

3. Acute tubular acute renal failure (ARF) except
A. Uraemia B. ↑ H$^+$ concentration
C. ↑ Ca^{++} D. ↑ K$^+$

4. Urine of low specific gravity is obtained in
A. B. Uraemia
C. B. Massive proteinuria
D. Severe dehydration

5. Broad casts are found in
A. Acute glomerulonephritis B. Myxoedema
C. Cirrhosis of liver D. Lymphoma

49. Which of the following is not seen in haemolytic-uraemic syndrome
A. Analgesic nephropathy D. Chronic renal failure (CRF)

6. Fruity odour in urine is found in all except
A. Urinary tract infection (UTI) B. Diabetic ketoacidosis
C. Alkaptonuria D. Chyluria

7. Most beneficial drug in enuresis is
A. D.

50. All the following drugs produce methaemoglobinaemia except
A. Chlorpromazine B. Phenacetin
A. Sodium nitroprusside D. Trimipramine

8. Urine osmolarity of 150 compared with plasma is found to be < 10 in
A. Membranous nephropathy
B. Minimal lesion nephropathy

51. Henoch-Schonlein purpura is not associated with
A. Membranous nephropathy
B. Minimal lesion nephropathy
C. Focal glomerulosclerosis
D. Mesangial proliferative nephropathy
D. Acute diffuse glomerulonephritis

64. The ESR may be 'zero' in

A. Old age
B. Vasculitis
C. Afibrinogenaemia
D. SLE

65. Which of the following is not recognised to be an acute phase reactant

A. Alpha fetoprotein
B. Orosomucoid
C. Caeruloplasmin
D. Haptoglobulin

66. All are examples of congenital cyanotic heart disease *except*

A. Ebstein's anomaly
B. Anomalous origin of coronary artery
C. Fallot's tetralogy
D. Single ventricle

67. Lutembacher's syndrome is

A. ASD plus AI
B. VSD plus MS
C. ASD plus MI
D. ASD plus MS

68. Differential diagnoses of ASD at the bedside are all *except*

A. Total anomalous pulmonary venous connection (TAPVC)
B. Idiopathic pulmonary artery dilatation
C. PDA
D. Pulmonary stenosis

69. 'Fallot's pentalogy' is Fallot's tetralogy plus

A. ASD
B. PDA
C. Associated LVH
D. AS

70. All are commonly associated with ASD *except*

A. Ellis-van Creveld syndrome
B. Holt-Oram syndrome
C. Down's syndrome
D. Trisomy 18

71. Coarctation of aorta may be associated with all *except*

A. Polycystic kidney
B. Berry aneurysm
C. Bicuspid aortic valve
D. Aortic arch syndrome

72. Commonest congenital heart disease is

A. ASD
B. VSD
C. Bicuspid aortic valve
D. Fallot's tetralogy

Ans: 64-C 65-A 66-B 67-D 68-C 69-A 70-D 71-D 72-C

110. During cardiopulmonary resuscitation, external defibrillation by DC shock is done with

    A. 50 Joules
    C. 200 Joules
    D. 400 Joules

111. Differential cyanosis is found in

    A. Fallot's tetralogy
    C. VSD
    B. Transposition of great vessels
    D. Ebstein's anomaly

112. Very close differential diagnosis of constrictive pericarditis at the bedside is

    A. Congestive cardiac failure
    C. Left ventricular failure
    B. Superior mediastinal syndrome
    D. Cirrhosis of liver

113. All are features of pericardial tamponade *except*

    A. Orthopnoea
    C. Hypotension
    B. Pulsatile liver
    D. Raised JVP

114. Acute myocardial infarction of posterior wall of left ventricle will show in the ECG

    A. Deep Q waves in V_{1-6}
    B. ST depression and tall R wave in V_{1-4}
    C. ST elevation in II, III, aVF
    D. ST elevation in I, aVL, V_6

115. Which one of the following is false regarding Austin Flint murmur

    A. Found in severe AI
    C. Mid-diastolic murmur
    B. Having loud S_1
    D. Absence of thrill

116. Acute subendocardial infarction will have ECG finding

    A. Prominent ST elevation
    B. Deep Q wave
    C. Deep symmetrical T wave inversion
    D. Height of R wave maximum in V_6

117. 'Auscultatory gap' in BP measurement is

    A. Present in all hypertensives
    C. Related to diastolic BP
    B. Should be ignored
    D. As a result of venous distension

118. All of the following are common arrhythmias developing from AMI *except*

    A. Sinus arrhythmia
    B. Ventricular tachycardia
    C. Wenckebach heart block
    D. Accelerated idioventricular rhythm

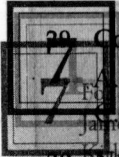

29. Commonest histological variety of nephrotic syndrome in adult is

   A. Minimal lesion   B. Focal glomerulosclerosis

   C. Mesangial proliferative   D. Membranous

30. Normal urinary osmolality in mOsm ... approximately

   A. 150–200

   C. 400–700   D. 800–950

31. Which of the following is false regarding Tamm-Horsfall mucoprotein

   A. Schumm test is done in detecting it

   B. Does not arise from plasma

   C. Secreted by renal tubules

   D. Glycoprotein in nature

32. All of the following causes intravascular haemolysis except

   A. Hepatitis B

   C. Kala-azar   D. Pneumococcus

33. Acute tubular necrosis is found in all except

   A. Weil's disease   B. Rhabdomyolysis

   C. ...   D. Cisplatin-induced

34. Isolated haematuria is not found in

   A. Renal tuberculosis   B. Papillary necrosis

   C. ...   D. Sickle-cell nephropathy

35. Complement C_3 is characteristically low in all except

   B. SLE

   C. Focal glomerulosclerosis

   D. Post-streptococcal glomerulonephritis

36. Which of the following metal is not responsible for development of nephrotic syndrome

   A. Mercury   B. Iron

   C. Gold

37. Which of the following common cause acute kidney injury

   A. Rheumatoid arthritis

   C. Lithium

8. Serum vitamin B12 level is increased in
   A. Pernicious anaemia
   B. di Guglielmo's disease
   C. Chronic myeloid leukaemia
   D. Hereditary ...

8.38. Nephrotic syndrome may be associated with hypertension in all except
   D. Subacute bacterial endocarditis (SBE)

9. Post-splenectomy peripheral blood picture does not contain
   A. Howell-Jolly bodies
   B. ...
   C. ...
   D. ...

39. Which is false regarding Berger's disease
   A. ...
   C. Recurrent haematuria

10. Commonest cause of jaundice in thalassaemia is
   A. Viral hepatitis
   B. Drug
   C. ...
   D. Haemolysis

40. Diabetes mellitus complicated by nephrotic syndrome has all the following features except

11. Waldeyer's ring does not include
   A. Apical tonsils
   B. Submandibular glands
   C. Adenoids
   D. Lingual tonsils

12. Which of the following anaemia is associated with splenomegaly

41. Commonest cause of renal vein thrombosis in a child is

13. Haemoglobin A2 contains
   A. α2γ2
   B. α2δ2
   C. α2β2
   D. ...

14. Leucocyte alkaline phosphatase (LAP) score is diminished in
   A. Sickle cell anaemia
   B. Lymphoma
   C. Paroxysmal nocturnal haemoglobinuria (PNH)
   D. Thalassaemia major

42. Haemolysis associated with renal failure is found in all except
   Accelerated hypertension should not have
   B. Arteriovenous nipping

15. Epitrochlear adenopathy may be produced by all except
   A. Secondary syphilis
   B. Tularaemia
   C. Sarcoidosis
   D. Leprosy

43. Commonest lesion in diabetic nephropathy is
   A. Diffuse glomerulosclerosis
   B. ...
   C. Chronic interstitial nephritis
   D. ...
   C. Arteriolar nephrosclerosis

16. All of the following may cause pain in abdomen in thalassaemia major except

44. Which is false regarding Goodpasture's disease
   A. Vasculitis
   B. Pulmonary haemorrhage
   C. Glomerulonephritis
   D. Antibody to glomerular basement membrane antigen

Ans. 8-C 9-D 10-D 11-B 12-C 13-C 14-C 15-D 16-A
Ans. 38-C 39-D 40-D 41-B 42-C 43-A 44-D

100. **Which of the following is not advocated in the treatment of acute pulmonary oedema**
    A. Frusemide
    B. Morphine
    C. Trendelenburg position
    D. Rotating tourniquets

101. **K...**
    A. Hypertrophic cardiomyopathy
    B. Right ventricular infarction
    C. ...
    D. ...

102. **All are class I antiarrhythmic drugs except**
    A. Disopyramide
    B. ...
    C. Verapamil
    D. Quinidine

103. **Cardiac involvement is absent in**
    A. Facio-scapulo-humeral dystrophy
    B. Myotonic dystrophy
    C. Duchenne type muscular dystrophy
    D. Friedreich's ataxia

104. **All of the following may have unilateral clubbing except**
    A. Tophaceous gout
    B. ...
    C. Sarcoidosis

105. **Digitalis toxicity is precipitated by ... except**
    A. Old age
    B. Hypokalaemia
    C. Renal failure
    D. Hepatic encephalopathy

106. **Cannon wave in the neck vein is seen in**
    A. Complete heart block
    B. Constrictive pericarditis
    C. Tricuspid incompetence
    D. Right atrial myxoma

107. **Left ventricular hypertrophy is associated with**
    A. AS
    B. AI
    C. MS
    D. ...

108. **Which of the following is ... constrictive pericarditis**
    A. Pulmonary oedema
    B. Raised JVP
    C. Ascites
    D. Pulsus paradoxus

109. **Prolonged QT interval ... except**
    A. Quinidine therapy
    B. ... hypothermia
    C. Vagal stimulation
    D. ...

ORIENT BLACKSWAN PRIVATE LIMITED

Registered Office
3-6-752 Himayatnagar, Hyderabad 500 029 (A.P.), India
E-mail: centraloffice@orientblackswan.com

Other Offices
Bangalore, Bhopal, Bhubaneshwar, Chennai,
Ernakulam, Guwahati, Hyderabad, Jaipur, Kolkata,
Lucknow, Mumbai, New Delhi, Patna

© Orient Blackswan Private Limited 2010
First Published 2010
Revised Edition 2012

ISBN 978 81 250 4795 7

Typeset by
Le Studio Graphique, Gurgaon 122 001
in Adobe Jenson Pro 11/13.2

Printed at
Shri Balaji Printers
Delhi

Published by
Orient Blackswan Private Limited
1/24 Asaf Ali Road
New Delhi 110 002
E-mail: delhi@orientblackswan.com

146. **Which of the following cardioselective beta-blockers is used in heart failure**

    A. Carvedilol   B. Atenolol
    C. Labetalol   D. Pindolol

147. **Which one is false regarding the presence of ejection click**

    A. Occurs immediately after S_1
    B. Stenosis is severe
    C. Presence indicates stenosis at valvular level
    D. Sharp and high-pitched clicking sound

148. **Congestive cardiac failure may be seen in all *except***

    A. Fallot's tetralogy
    C. PDA   D. Coarctation of aorta

149. **Treatment by heparin is best monitored by**

    A. Prothrombin time (PT)
    B. Clotting time (CT)
    C. Activated partial thromboplastin time (APTT)
    D. Fibrin degradation products

150. **Major cardiovascular manifestation in cri-du-chat syndrome is**

    A. Bicuspid aortic valve   B. VSD
    C. PDA   D. Dextrocardia

151. **'Nitrate tolerance' developing as a result of treating ischaemic heart disease by mononitrates is prevented by**

    A. Twice daily dosage schedule   B. Night-time single dosage
    C. Eccentric dosage schedule   D. Morning-time single dosage

152. **All of the following may produce hemiplegia by cerebral embolism *except***

    A. Mitral valve prolapse
    B. Atrial fibrillation
    C. Subacute bacterial endocarditis
    D. Right atrial myxoma

153. **Drug of choice in acute management of PSVT is**

    A. Amiodarone   B. Verapramil
    C. Metoprolol   D. Adenosine

154. **Which of the following gives rise to pulsation at the back**

    A. Coarctation of aorta   B. Budd-Chiari syndrome
    C. Hyperkinetic circulatory states   D. Aortic aneurysm

Ans: 146-A 147-B 148-A 149-A 150-B 151-C 152-D 153-D 154-A

105. All are examples of hypoplastic anaemia *except*
A. Hepatitis B-induced
B. Paroxysmal nocturnal haemoglobinuria
C. Systemic lupus erythematosus
D. Paroxysmal cold haemoglobinuria

106. Which of the following is not true regarding features of hyperviscosity
A. Fluctuating consciousness
B. Hyponatraemia
C. Central cyanosis
D. Thrombotic episodes

107. A patient with nephrocalcinosis, hyperchloraemic acidosis and alkaline urine is suffering from
A. Distal renal tubular acidosis
B. Nephrogenic diabetes insipidus
C. Proximal renal tubular acidosis
D. Vitamin D resistant rickets

108. Giant lysosomal granules in granulocytes associated with albinism is known in
A. Chédiak-Higashi syndrome
B. Diabetes mellitus
C. ... syndrome
D. Niemann-Pick disease

109. Immunoproliferative small intestinal disease (IPSID) is a variety of
A. Intestinal lymphoma
B. GI complication of AIDS
C. Adenocarcinoma
D. Carcinoid tumours

110. HAM test (acid serum test) is positive in
A. G6PD deficiency
B. ...
C. Paroxysmal nocturnal haemoglobinuria
D. ...

111. Erythropoietin is secreted from all of the following tumours *except*
A. Renal cell carcinoma
B. ...
C. ...
D. Cerebellar haemangioblastoma

112. Migratory thrombophlebitis is commonly seen with
A. Prepancreatic carcinoma
B. Bronchogenic carcinoma
C. Hepatoma
D. Carcinoma of the pancreas

113. Multiple myeloma does not feature
71. Which does not produce 'sterile pyuria'
  A. Pregnancy
  A. Intraseptal emphysema   B. Uric acid
  B. Hyperglobulinaemia   D. ↑ Phosphate
  B. Cyclophosphamide administration
  C. Curry's proteus

114. Which is not an example of microangiopathic haemolytic anaemia
  A. Paroxysmal ... haemoglobinuria
  B. Thrombotic thrombocytopenic purpura   B. *Staphylococcus*
  C. Disseminated intravascular coagulation
72. Rapidly progressive glomerulonephritis is not produced as a result of
  A. Dexamethasone
  D. Haemolytic uraemic syndrome
  B. Post-streptococcal glomerulonephritis

115. Leucoerythroblastic blood picture may be seen in all *except*
  A. Myelofibrosis
  A. Wegener's granulomatosis   B. Honeycomb lung
  B. Myelophthisic anaemia   B. Gaucher's disease
73. ... reliable ... test in urine is found in all *except*

116. Transitional myeloproliferative disorder is ... commonly seen in association with ... disorder ... homocystinuria commonly
74. All are true of dialysis dementia *except*
  A. Down's syndrome   B. Hyperventilation
  A. Raised intracranial tension   B. Myoclonus
  C. Ataxia telangiectasia
  D. Related to aluminium toxicity

75. Each kidney contains approximately
  A. 1 lakh nephrons   B. 10 lakh nephrons
117. Total serum LDH is not raised in
  C. 1 million nephrons   D. 10 million nephrons
  C. Haemolysis   D. Crush injury

76. Which is true in prerenal azotaemia
118. Sezary syndrome is
  A. Urinary Na concentration >20 mmol/l

77. Renal biopsy is contraindicated in all *except*
119. ... renal ... disease does not include

78. Renal tubular acidosis is not seen in

79. Commonest organism producing acute pyelonephritis is
  B. *E. coli*
  C. *Streptococcus*   D. *Klebsiella*

136. Which of the following is not a side effect of amiodarone

A.
C.

137. Sycophant with the associated possibilities

A.
B.
C.
D.

138. Compression of the feeding artery abruptly reduces the heart rate in arteriovenous fistula is

A.
C.

139. Pulmonary regurgitation is never associated with

A.
C.

140. Hyperkalaemia arrests the heart in

A.
C.

141. The drug contraindicated in pregnancy-induced hypertension is

A. Hydralazine   B. Enalapril

C. Methyldopa   Labetalol

142. Reversed splitting of S_2 is found in

A. LBBB   B. RBBB

C. Left ventricular pacing   D. Aortic regurgitation

143. All

A.
C.

144. Jane

A.

145. P

A. Radial   B. Brachial

C. Femoral   D. Any of the above

184. High-volume double-peaked pulse is found in all *except*

    A. AI   B. IHSS

    C. AS with AI   D. MI

185. Boot-shaped heart with oilgaemic lung fields is found in

    A.   B.

    C. Coarctation of aorta   D. Transposition of great vessels

186. Exercise tolerance test (TMT) is absolutely contraindicated in

    A. Aortic stenosis   B. Buerger's disease

    C. Unstable angina   D. Coarctation of aorta

187. Osler's node is classically seen in

    A.

188.

189. Commonest heart valve abnormality revealed after AMI is

    A. AI   B. MI

    C. AS   D. MS

190. Which of the following heart sounds occurs shortly after S_1

    A. Ejection click

    B. Opening snap

    C. Tumour plop in atrial myxoma

    D. Pericardial knock

191. Which of the following is not a natural vasodilator

    A. Bradykinin   B. Histamine

    C. Endothelin   D. Nitric oxide

192. Pseudoclaudication is due to compression of

    A. Inferior vena cava   B. Cauda equina

    C. Femoral artery   D. Popliteal artery

Ans: 184-D 185-B 186-A 187-C 188-C 189-B 190-A 191-C 192-B

97. Wilms' tumour is characterised by all except
A. Renal lump with smooth surface
B. Haematuria
C. Pain abdomen
D. Commonest renal malignancy

98. Serum urea and creatinine remain normal in
A. Hepatorenal syndrome
B. Haemolytic-uraemic syndrome
C. Hydronephrosis
D. Acute renal failure

99. All of the following are complications of chronic pyelonephritis except
A. Chronic renal failure
B. Septicaemia
C. Renal calculus cyst
D. Hypertension

100. Transient deafness is most commonly associated with
A. Ethacrynic acid
B. Spironolactone
C. Hydrochlorthiazide
D. Bumetanide

101. The urine in obligatory diuresis following relief of urinary obstruction is
A. concentrated
B. more than 60 mM sodium
C. ...
D. ...

102. Blood level of all raises in ARF except
A. ...
B. ...
C. ...
D. ...

103. Which of the following is not added to urine by tubular secretion
A. K
B. Urea
C. Creatinine
D. ...

104. 'Rugger jersey spine' is seen in
A. Ochronosis
B. Chronic renal failure
C. ...
D. Hypoparathyroidism

105. X-ray pelvis shows iliac horns in
A. Fabry's disease
B. Nail-patella syndrome
C. Alport's syndrome
D. Medullary sponge kidney

68. Which of the following is false in primary pulmonary tuberculosis
A. ...
B. ...
C. ... Fibrosis
D. Pleural effusion

69. All of the following may complicate bone marrow transplantation except
A. Cataract formation
B. Leucoencephalopathy
C. Cardiomyopathy
D. Emphysema

70. Palpable purpura is seen in
A. Idiopathic thrombocytopenic purpura
B. Quinine associated thrombocytopenia
C. Heparin associated thrombocytopenia
D. Leucocytoclastic vasculitis

71. Which isolated coagulation factor deficiency causes thrombosis
A. Factor X
B. Factor VII
C. ...
D. ...

72. Incorrect statement in pernicious anaemia is
A. Hyperchlorhydria
B. premature greying of hair
C. intrinsic factor antibody in 60% patients
D. Gastric polyp may develop

73. Which of the following is not found in polycythaemia vera
A. Increased RBC mass
B. ...
C. Markedly hypocellular marrow
D. Thrombocytopenia

74. Busulfan therapy may lead to all except
A. Hyperpigmentation
B. Chronic bone marrow suppression
C. Optic neuritis
D. Pulmonary fibrosis

75. Hand-Schüller-Christian disease does not have
A. Hypercholesterolaemia
B. Exophthalmos
C. Guillain-Barré syndrome
D. Hepatosplenomegaly

76. ↑ Serum iron and ↓ iron-binding capacity is a feature of
A. ...
B. Sideroblastic anaemia
C. Alcoholic liver disease
D. Thalassaemia major

Ans: 97-D 98-C 99-B 100-A 101-C 102-C 103-B 104-B 105-B
Ans: 68-B 69-D 70-D 71-D 72-A 73-C 74-C 75-A 76-B

106. Green urine is seen in
A. Pseudomonas infection
B.
C. Oxalate poisoning
D.

77. Alopecia mucinosa may be seen in
A.
B. Alcaptonuria
C. Mycosis fungoides
D.

107. Hypernephroma is associated with all except
A. High incidence of hypertension
B. Renal vein thrombosis
C. Haematuria
D. Polycythaemia

78. Disseminated intravascular coagulation (DIC) may be seen in all except
A.
B. Rocky Mountain spotted fever
C.
D. Diabetes mellitus

108. All of these may give rise to Fanconi's syndrome except
A. Wilson's disease
B. Galactosaemia
C.
D.

79. Acanthosis nigricans may be associated with all except
A. Diabetes mellitus
B.
C. Carcinoma of the stomach
D. Ulcerative colitis

109. Chronic anaemia may lead to all except
A.
B.
C.
D.

80.
A.
B.
C.
D.

110. Non-Hodgkin's lymphoma is classified under the name of
A.
B.
C.
D.

81.
A.
B.
C.
D.

111. Prognosis of transplant is excellent
A. Acute cellular rejection
B.
C.
D.

82.
A.
B.
C.
D.

112. Which of all is correct
A.
B.
C.
D.

83.
A.
B.
C.
D.

113. All of the following can present as nephritic/nephrotic syndrome except
A.
B.
C.
D.

84. All are features of tropical pulmonary eosinophilia except
A. Eosinophilia >3000/mm³
B. Miliary mottling in chest X-ray
C. High IgE level
D. Response to albendazole therapy

114. Bosselation is recognised by
A.
B.
C.
D.

85. Hepatosplenomegaly with lymphadenopathy is found in all except
A. Acute lymphatic leukaemia
B.
C. Chronic myeloid leukaemia
D. Disseminated tuberculosis

115. IgA nephropathy commonly presents with
A. Systemic hypertension
B. Acute renal failure
C. Haematuria
D. Nephrotic syndrome

86. Iron transport protein is
A. Ceruloplasmin
B. Ferritin
C. Haptoglobin
D. Transferrin

176. When a patient of unstable angina worsens by nitroglycerine, the diagnosis is
    A. MS
    B. Left main coronary artery stenosis
    C. MI
    D. Idiopathic subaortic stenosis

177. Increased PR interval is observed in
    A. AV nodal rhythm   B. First degee heart block
    C. W-P-W syndrome   D. Low atrial rhythm

178. Pulmonary capillary wedge pressure is increased in all *except*
    A. Right ventricular infarction
    B. Cardiac tamponade
    C. Acute mitral regurgitation
    D. Cardiogenic shock due to myocardial dysfunction

179. Which of the following does not produce continuous murmur over the chest
    A. Ruptured sinus of Valsalva   B. Patent ductus arteriosus
    C. Aortopulmonary window   D. Ventricular septal defect

180. Inverted P-wave in lead I, upright P-wave in aVR and gradual diminution of the height of R-waves in precordial leads are found in
    A. Emphysema
    B. Faulty interchange of right and left arm electrode
    C. Dextrocardia
    D. ECG taken at height of deep inspiration

181. Commonest cause of displacement of apex beat is
    A. Left ventricular hypertrophy B. Thoracic deformity
    C. Cardiomyopathy   D. Right ventricular hypertrophy

182. Graham Steell murmur is found in
    A. Severe pulmonary hypertension
    B. Subacute bacterial endocarditis
    C. Idiopathic hypertrophic subaortic stenosis (IHSS)
    D. Tricuspid atresia

183. Drug to be avoided in hypertensive encephalopathy
    A. Labetalol   B. Diazoxide
    C. Methyldopa   D. Sodium nitroprusside

Ans: 176-D 177-B 178-A 179-D 180-C 181-B 182-A 183-C

125. **WBC casts in urine are suggestive of all *except***

A. Transplant rejection
B. Rapidly progressive glomerulonephritis
C. Interstitial nephritis
D. Pyelonephritis

126. **Struvite stone are usually result of urinary infection by**

A. *Staphylococcus*   B. *Proteus*
C. *Pseudomonas*   D. *Klebsiella*

127. **Renal tubular acidosis may be due to**

A. Methoxyflurane   B. Streptozotocin
C. Captopril   D. Probenecid

128. **Regarding erythropoietin therapy in CRF, which is not correct**

A. Patients with ferritin level 50–100 µg/l respond well
B. Average dosage is 50 U/kg, IV, thrice weekly
C. During treatment, haemoglobin should not cross 12 g/dl
D. Subcutaneous administration may give rise to pure red cell aplasia

129. **Acute tubular necrosis may be caused by all of the following *except***

A. Hepatorenal syndrome   B. Systemic hypertension
C. Acute pancreatitis   D. Congestive cardiac failure

130. **Which of the following is false in nephritic-nephrotic syndrome**

A. Moderate haematuria and moderate proteinuria are common
B. A majority of patients terminate into end-stage renal disease
C. SLE is a common aetiology
D. Systemic hypertension is rare

1. **Schumm test is done to detect**
   A. Haptoglobin
   B. Methaemalbumin
   C. Cirtulline
   D. Haemopexin

2. **All of the following are seen in intravascular haemolysis** *except*
   A. High urinary urobilinogen
   B. Reticulocytosis
   C. High plasma haemopexin
   D. High urinary haemosiderin

3. **Which of the following is false regarding Philadelphia chromosome**
   A. Shortening of long arm of chromosome G22
   B. Philadelphia -ve cases have bad prognosis
   C. Diagnostic of CML
   D. Found in lymphocytes

4. **Auer rods are found in**
   A. Acute myeloid leukaemia (AML)
   B. Blast crisis of CML
   C. Acute lymphatic leukaemia (ALL)
   D. Blast crisis of CLL

5. **'Cast iron spleen' is classically found in**
   A. Tropical splenomegaly syndrome
   B. Myelofibrosis
   C. Chronic myeloid leukaemia (CML)
   D. Thalassaemia major

6. **Which of the following does not produce iron-overload in body**
   A. Chronic haemodialysis
   B. Pernicious anaemia
   C. Alcoholic liver disease
   D. Sideroblastic anaemia

7. **Pseudolymphoma may be produced by all** *except*
   A. Cyclosporine
   B. Primidone
   C. Lithium
   D. Phenytoin

Ans: 1-B 2-C 3-D 4-A 5-C 6-B 7-C

8. Serum vitamin B_{12} level is increased in
   A. Pernicious anaemia
   B. di Guglielmo's disease
   C. Chronic myeloid leukaemia
   D. Hereditary orotic aciduria

9. Post-splenectomy peripheral blood picture does not contain
   A. Howell-Jolly bodies   B. Heinz bodies
   C. Target cells   D. Doehle bodies

10. Commonest cause of jaundice in thalassaemia is
   A. Viral hepatitis C
   B. Iron deposition in liver
   C. Viral hepatitis B
   D. Haemolysis

11. Waldeyer's ring does not include
   A. Faucal tonsils   B. Submandibular glands
   C. Adenoids   D. Lingual tonsils

12. Which of the following anaemias is associated with splenomegaly
   A. Chronic renal failure   B. Aplastic anaemia
   C. Hereditary spherocytosis D. Sickle-cell anaemia

13. Haemoglobin A_2 is
   A. $\alpha_2 \gamma_2$ B. δ_2
   C. $\alpha_2 \delta_2$ C. $\alpha_2 \beta_2$

14. Leucocyte alkaline phosphatase (LAP) score is diminished in
   A. Sickle-cell anaemia
   B. Lymphoma
   C. Paroxysmal nocturnal haemoglobinuria (PNH)
   D. Thalassaemia major

15. Epitrochlear adenopathy may be produced by all except
   A. Secondary syphilis   B. Tularaemia
   C. Sarcoidosis   D. Leprosy

16. All of the following may cause pain abdomen in thalassaemia major except
   A. Vasculitis
   B. Splenic infarction
   C. Dragging pain due to huge splenomegaly
   D. Pigment stone-induced biliary colic

Ans: 8-C 9-D 10-D 11-B 12-C 13-C 14-C 15-D 16-A

17. Which of the following does not have target cells in peripheral blood
    A. Lymphoma
    B. Cholestatic jaundice
    C. Thalassaemia
    D. Iron deficiency anaemia

18. Virchow's node receives lymphatics from all *except*
    A. Testes
    B. Stomach
    C. Prostate
    D. Breast (left)

19. Reed-Sternberg cell is found in all *except*
    A. Infectious mononucleosis
    B. Hodgkin's disease
    C. Kaposi's sarcoma
    D. Breast carcinoma

20. All of the following produce microcytic anaemia *except*
    A. Sideroblastic anaemia
    B. Thalassaemia
    C. Pernicious anaemia
    D. Lead poisoning

21. 'Suggilations' are haemorrhagic spots in the size of
    A. 1–2 mm in diameter
    B. 2–5 mm in diameter
    C. > 10 mm in diameter
    D. > 20 mm in diameter

22. All of the following may produce agranulocytosis *except*
    A. Methyldopa
    B. Methimazole
    C. Gold salts
    D. Chloramphenicol

23. Basophilia is classically found in
    A. Non-Hodgkin's lymphoma
    B. Hodgkin's disease
    C. Melanoma
    D. Chronic myeloid leukaemia

24. Which of the following is not a myelodysplastic syndrome (MDS)
    A. Refractory anaemia with ring sideroblasts
    B. Refractory anaemia with excess of blasts
    C. Acute myelomonocytic leukaemia
    D. Refractory anaemia

25. Eosinophilia is caused by all *except*
    A. Oxyphenbutazone
    B. Iodides
    C. Nitrofurantoin
    D. Sulphonamides

26. **Leucocyte alkaline phosphatase (LAP) score is high in all** *except*
   A. Chronic myeloid leukaemia
   B. Polycythaemia vera
   C. After steroid administration
   D. Myelosclerosis

27. **Basophilic stippling is classically seen in**
   A. Chronic myeloid leukaemia B. Myelosclerosis
   C. Chronic lead poisoning   D. Iron deficiency anaemia

28. **Chloroma is found in**
   A. Acute lymphatic leukaemia (ALL)
   B. Chronic myeloid leukaemia (CML)
   C. Acute myeloid leukaemia (AML)
   D. Non-Hodgkin's lymphoma (NHL)

29. **Which of the following is not a myeloproliferative disorder**
   A. Chronic myeloid leukaemia B. Polycythaemia vera
   C. Essential thrombocytopenia D. Myeloid metaplasia

30. **↑ Fe and normal TIBC are found in**
   A. Thalassaemia major   B. Haemosiderosis
   C. Rheumatoid arthritis   D. Disseminated malignancy

31. **Non-thrombocytopenic purpura is seen in all** *except*
   A. Vasculitis
   B. Uraemia
   C. Hereditary haemorrhagic telangiectasis
   D. SLE

32. **Pelger-Huet anomaly is**
   A. Hereditary hypersegmentation of neutrophils
   B. Presence of Doehle bodies in neutrophils
   C. Faulty maturation of platelets
   D. Hereditary hyposegmentation of neutrophils

33. **Intravascular half-life of factor VIII is**
   A. 5 hours   B. 12 hours
   C. 1–3 days   D. 4–5 days

34. **Gum bleeding is characteristic of all** *except*
   A. Chronic phenytoin therapy B. Aplastic anaemia
   C. Scurvy   D. Haemophilia

Ans: 26-A 27-C 28-C 29-C 30-A 31-D 32-D 33-B 34-A

35. **Which of the following is not true in thrombasthenia**

    A. Prolonged bleeding time   B. Normal platelet count
    C. Platelet aggregation defect   D. Prolonged clotting time

36. **Which of the following is not associated with hypersplenism**

    A. Splenomegaly
    B. Hypocellular bone marrow
    C. Pancytopenia
    D. Reversibility by splenectomy

37. **Splenectomy is virtually curative in**

    A. G6PD deficiency
    B. Idiopathic thrombocytopenic purpura (ITP)
    C. Thalassaemia
    D. Hereditary spherocytosis

38. **In chronic granulomatous disease, which is false**

    A. Prone to infection by staphylococci
    B. Neutrophil count is normal
    C. Difficulty in phagocytosis
    D. Diagnosed by amount of nitroblue tetrazolium reduction

39. **Thymoma may be associated with all of the following** *except*

    A. Cushing's syndrome   B. Hypergammaglobulinaemia
    C. Myasthenia gravis   D. Pure red cell aplasia

40. **Red cell osmotic fragility is increased in**

    A. Thalassaemia major   B. Hereditary spherocytosis
    C. Hb C disease   D. Iron deficiency anaemia

41. **Plummer-Vinson syndrome is not associated with**

    A. Angular stomatitis   B. Splenomegaly
    C. Clubbing   D. Post-cricoid web

42. **Warm-antibody mediated haemolysis is not found in**

    A. SLE
    B. Infectious mononucleosis
    C. Non-Hodgkin's lymphoma
    D. Chronic lymphatic leukaemia

43. **Haemolytic anaemia is not produced by**

    A. Penicillin   B. Lithium
    C. Quinidine   D. Methyldopa

Ans: 35-D 36-B 37-D 38-C 39-B 40-B 41-C 42-B 43-B

44. **All of the following are true in paroxysmal nocturnal haemoglobinuria (PNH)** *except*

    A. Low leucocyte alkaline phosphatase
    B. Elevated LDH
    C. Positive acidified serum lysis (HAM) test
    D. Elevated red cell acetylcholinesterase

45. **Sideroblastic anaemia may be treated by all** *except*

    A. Pyridoxine B. Hydroxyurea
    C. Desferrioxamine D. Androgens

46. **Which of the following is not true in paroxysmal cold haemoglobinuria**

    A. Associated with mycoplasma infection
    B. IgG antibody-mediated
    C. Precipitated by exposure to cold
    D. Not a cold agglutinin disease

47. **Myelophthisic anaemia is characterised by all** *except*

    A. Leucoerythroblastic blood picture
    B. Caused by disseminated malignancy
    C. Basophilic stippling
    D. Neutropenia

48. **Spur cell anaemia is seen in**

    A. Uraemia B. Myxoedema
    C. Cirrhosis of liver D. Lymphoma

49. **Which of the following is not seen in haemolytic-uraemic syndrome**

    A. Positive Coombs test
    B. Thrombocytopenia
    C. High creatinine level
    D. Hypofibrinogenaemia

50. **All the following drugs produce methaemoglobinaemia** *except*

    A. Amyl nitrite B. Phenacetin
    C. Sodium nitroprusside D. Hydralazine

51. **Henoch-Schönlein purpura is not associated with**

    A. Thrombocytopenia
    B. Palpable purpura
    C. Intussusception
    D. Acute diffuse glomerulonephritis

Ans: 44-D 45-B 46-A 47-D 48-C 49-A 50-D 51-A

52. **Which of the following is false about methaemoglobinaemia**
    A. If exceeds >0.5 g/dl, produces cyanotic hue
    B. Hereditary variety is due to deficiency of methaemoglobin reductase
    C. Normal red cells contain <1% methaemoglobin
    D. Oral or I.V. methylene blue is treatment of choice

53. **Conditions resistant to malaria are all *except***
    A. Duffy -ve blood group   B. HbC disease
    C. Sickle-cell disease   D. Thalassaemia major

54. **The outstanding feature of idiopathic thrombocytopenic purpura (ITP) is**
    A. Fever   B. Gum bleeding
    C. Moderate splenomegaly   D. Presence of sternal tenderness

55. **Vitamin C is used in low dose (3 mg/kg) in thalassaemia major as in high dose it produces**
    A. Nephrotoxicity   B. Cardiotoxicity
    C. Hepatotoxicity   D. Neurotoxicity

56. **Which of the following is not seen in sickle-cell anaemia**
    A. Isosthenuria
    B. Leg ulcers
    C. Leucopenia
    D. Corkscrew vessel in bulbar conjunctiva

57. **Thrombocytopenia is absent in**
    A. Disseminated intravascular coagulation
    B. Wiskott-Aldrich syndrome
    C. Henoch-Schonlein purpura
    D. Myelosclerosis

58. **Sickle-cell anaemia is associated with**
    A. Cerebral embolism
    B. High ESR
    C. Fishmouth vertebrae
    D. Diastolic murmur over precordium

59. **Cooley's anaemia is**
    A. Sickle-cell anaemia   B. Megaloblastic anaemia
    C. Thalassaemia major   D. Aplastic anaemia

Ans: 52-A 53-D 54-B 55-B 56-C 57-C 58-C 59-C

60. **Presence of anaemia, jaundice and splenomegaly with increased mean corpuscular haemoglobin concentration (MCHC) is seen in**
    A. Cirrhosis of liver
    B. Thalassaemia major
    C. Paroxysmal nocturnal haemoglobinuria (PNH)
    D. Hereditary spherocytosis

61. **Which of the following is false in hereditary haemorrhagic telangiectasis**
    A. Telangiectasia in skin and mucous membrane
    B. Telangiectasia does not blanch on pressure
    C. May have haematemesis
    D. Positive familial pattern

62. **Plasmapheresis may be done in all *except***
    A. Cryoglobulinaemia
    B. Goodpasture's disease
    C. Hypoplastic anaemia
    D. Myasthenia gravis

63. **vW antigen level is increased in**
    A. Pregnancy
    B. Lymphoma
    C. von Willebrand disease
    D. Multiple myeloma

64. **Which of the following is not found in eosinophilic granuloma**
    A. Eosinophilia
    B. Osteolytic lesions in bone
    C. Affection in young adults
    D. Absence of systemic manifestations

65. **Circulating anticoagulants are found in**
    A. Hairy cell leukaemia
    B. SLE
    C. Multiple myeloma
    D. Dermatomyositis

66. **Which of the following is not true in thrombotic thrombocytopenic purpura**
    A. Fluctuating consciousness
    B. Coombs -ve haemolysis
    C. Fragmented platelets
    D. Early development of acute renal failure

67. **In polycythaemia vera, which is not true**
    A. Low level of erythropoietin
    B. High ESR
    C. Increased LAP score
    D. High serum vitamin B_{12} level

Ans: 60-D 61-B 62-C 63-A 64-A 65-B 66-C 67-B

68. **Which of the following is false in haemophilia**
    A. Normal prothrombin time
    B. von Willebrand antigens level is grossly diminished
    C. Increased partial thromboplastin time
    D. Absent factor VIII coagulant activity

69. **All of the following may complicate bone marrow transplantation** *except*
    A. Cataract formation
    B. Leucoencephalopathy
    C. Cardiomyopathy
    D. Emphysema

70. **Palpable purpura is seen in**
    A. Idiopathic thrombocytopenic purpura
    B. Quinine therapy
    C. Heparin-associated thrombocytopenia
    D. Leucocytoclastic vasculitis

71. **Which isolated coagulation factor deficiency causes thrombosis**
    A. Factor V
    B. Factor VII
    C. Factor XI
    D. Factor XII

72. **Incorrect statement in pernicious anaemia is**
    A. Hyperchlorhydria
    B. Premature greying of hair
    C. Anti-intrinsic factor antibody in 60% patients
    D. Gastric polyp may develop

73. **Which of the following is not true in polycythaemia vera**
    A. Increased RBC mass
    B. Markedly hypercellular marrow
    C. Thrombocytopenia
    D. Basophilia

74. **Busulfan therapy may lead to all** *except*
    A. Hyperpigmentation
    B. Pulmonary fibrosis
    C. Optic neuritis
    D. Bone marrow suppression

75. **Hand-Schüller-Christian disease does not have**
    A. Hypercholesterolaemia
    B. Exophthalmos
    C. Diabetes mellitus
    D. Hepatosplenomegaly

76. **↑ Serum iron and ↓ iron-binding capacity is a feature of**
    A. Hookworm infestation
    B. Sideroblastic anaemia
    C. Alcoholic liver disease
    D. Thalassaemia major

Ans: 68-B 69-D 70-D 71-D 72-A 73-C 74-C 75-A 76-B

77. **Alopecia mucinosa may be seen in**
    A. Mycosis fungoides
    B. Carcinoid syndrome
    C. Amyloidosis
    D. Pancreatic carcinoma

78. **Disseminated intravascular coagulation (DIG) may be seen in all** *except*
    A. Amniotic fluid embolism
    B. Rocky Mountain spotted fever
    C. Giant haemangioma
    D. Diabetes mellitus

79. **Acanthosis nigricans may be associated with all** *except*
    A. Diabetes mellitus
    B. Stein-Leventhal syndrome
    C. Carcinoma of the stomach
    D. Ulcerative colitis

80. **Thalassaemia major may be associated with all** *except*
    A. Cardiac arrhythmia
    B. Cardiac tamponade
    C. Congestive cardiac failure
    D. Cardiomegaly

81. **Non-Hodgkin's lymphoma is classified under the name of**
    A. Rye
    B. Ann Arbor
    C. Rappaport
    D. Dorothy Reed

82. **Macrocytic-hypochromic anaemia is found in**
    A. Iron deficiency anaemia
    B. Pregnancy
    C. Thalassaemia
    D. Pernicious anaemia

83. **Hess' capillary fragility test is positive in**
    A. Cushing's syndrome
    B. Idiopathic thrombocytopenic purpura
    C. Paraproteinaemias
    D. Vasculitis

84. **All are features of tropical pulmonary eosinophilia** *except*
    A. Eosinophilia >3000/mm^3
    B. Miliary mottling in chest X-ray
    C. High IgE level
    D. Response to albendazole therapy

85. **Hepatospenomegaly with lymphadenopathy is found in all** *except*
    A. Acute lymphatic leukaemia
    B. Lymphoma
    C. Chronic myeloid leukaemia
    D. Disseminated tuberculosis

86. **Iron transport protein is**
    A. Transcobalamin II
    B. Ferritin
    C. Haptoglobin
    D. Transferrin

Ans: 77-A 78-D 79-D 80-B 81-C 82-B 83-B 84-D 85-C 86-D

87. **Most effective treatment of polycythaemia vera is**
   A. Fresh frozen plasma   B. Splenectomy
   C. Phlebotomy   D. Exchange transfusion

88. **Commonest pathogen involved in sickle-cell anaemia-induced osteomyelitis is**
   A. *Salmonella*   B. *Streptococcus*
   C. *Nocardia*   D. *Staphylococcus*

89. **Which is not a vitamin K-dependent factor**
   A. Factor VIII   B. Factor VII
   C. Factor X   D. Factor II

90. **Eosinophilia is a feature of**
   A. Non-Hodgkin's lymphoma   B. Sickle-cell anaemia
   C. Hodgkin's disease   D. Haemophilia

91. **Which is a bad prognostic sign in Hodgkin's disease**
   A. Lymphocytopenia
   B. Thrombocytopenia
   C. Eosinophilia
   D. Reed-Sternberg cells in marrow

92. **Sickle-cell anaemia is not complicated by**
   A. Papillary necrosis   B. Pancreatitis
   C. Osteomyelitis   D. Congestive cardiac failure

93. **↓ iron and ↓ iron-binding capacity are seen in**
   A. Recurrent GI tract haemorrhage
   B. Intestinal resection
   C. Chronic infections
   D. Menorrhagia

94. **Best prognostic indicator in multiple myeloma is**
   A. Serum β_2 microglobulins
   B. Bence Jones protein in urine
   C. Number of plasma cells
   D. Serum calcium level in marrow

95. **All are true regarding midline granuloma *except***
   A. Pathological hallmark is non-caseating granuloma
   B. Produces perforation of nasal septum
   C. More common in men
   D. The treatment of choice is radiotherapy

Ans: 87-C 88-A 89-A 90-C 91-A 92-B 93-C 94-A 95-C

96. **Among the following, treatment of choice in hairy cell leukaemia is**
    A. Deoxycoformycin
    B. Corticosteroid
    C. Splenectomy
    D. Hydroxyurea

97. **Tumour lysis syndrome produces all *except***
    A. Hyperuricaemia
    B. Hyperkalaemia
    C. Hypercalcaemia
    D. Hyperphosphataemia

98. **Carcino-embryonic antigen is the tumour marker of**
    A. Ovarian carcinoma
    B. Hepatocellular carcinoma
    C. Bronchogenic carcinoma
    D. Colorectal carcinoma

99. **Platelet transfusion is not indicated in**
    A. Aplastic anaemia
    B. Uraemia with bleeding
    C. Disseminated intravascular coagulation
    D. Immunogenic thrombocytopenia

100. **Wiskott-Aldrich syndrome does not feature**
    A. Thrombocytopenia
    B. Haemolytic anaemia
    C. Eczema
    D. Repeated infections

101. **Waldenstrom's macroglobulinaemia commonly has all the features *except***
    A. Lymphadenopathy
    B. Hyperviscosity syndrome
    C. Renal failure
    D. Anaemia

102. **Best treatment modality in chronic myeloid leukaemia is**
    A. Hydroxyurea
    B. Allogenic bone marrow transplantation
    C. Interferon-α
    D. Radiotherapy

103. **Which is not true in relation to multiple myeloma**
    A. Hyperviscosity syndrome
    B. Renal failure
    C. Moderate splenomegaly
    D. Response to melphalan

104. **Autoimmune haemolytic anaemia is associated with**
    A. ALL
    B. CLL
    C. AML
    D. CML

Ans: 96-A 97-C 98-D 99-D 100-B 101-C 102-B 103-C 104-B

105. **All are examples of hypoplastic anaemia** *except*
    A. Hepatitis B-induced
    B. Paroxysmal nocturnal haemoglobinuria
    C. Systemic lupus erythematosus
    D. Paroxysmal cold haemoglobinuria

106. **Which of the following is not true regarding features of hyperviscosity syndrome**
    A. Fluctuating consciousness   B. Raynaud's phenomenon
    C. Central cyanosis   D. Thrombotic episodes

107. **Which of the following is contraindicated in polycythaemia vera**
    A. Hydroxyurea
    B. Chlorambucil
    C. Interferon-α
    D. Baby aspirin to prevent thrombosis

108. **Giant lysosomal granules in granulocytes associated with albinism is known as**
    A. May-Hegglin anomaly   B. Chediak-Higashi syndrome
    C. Schultz syndrome   D. Niemann-Pick disease

109. **Immunoproliferative small intestinal disease (IPSID) is a variety of**
    A. Intestinal lymphoma   B. GI complication of AIDS
    C. Adenocarcinoma   D. Carcinoid tumours

110. **HAM test (acid serum test) is positive in**
    A. G6PD deficiency
    B. Myelodysplastic syndrome
    C. Paroxysmal nocturnal haemoglobinuria
    D. Haemolytic-uraemic syndrome

111. **Erythropoietin is secreted from all of the following tumours** *except*
    A. Renal-cell carcinoma
    B. Phaeochromocytoma
    C. Cerebellar haemangioblastoma
    D. Oat-cell carcinoma of lung

112. **Migratory thrombophlebitis is commonly due to**
    A. Hepatocellular carcinoma   B. Bronchogenic carcinoma
    C. Hypernephroma   D. Carcinoma of the pancreas

Ans: 105-D 106-C 107-B 108-B 109-A 110-C 111-D 112-D

113. **Multiple myeloma does not feature**
    A. ↑ Calcium
    B. ↑ Uric acid
    C. Hyperglobulinaemia
    D. ↑ Phosphate

114. **Which is not an example of microangiopathic haemolytic anaemia**
    A. Paroxysmal cold haemoglobinuria
    B. Thrombotic thrombocytopenic purpura
    C. Disseminated intravascular coagulation
    D. Haemolytic-uraemic syndrome

115. **Leucoerythroblastic blood picture may be seen in all *except***
    A. Myelophthisic anaemia
    B. Gaucher's disease
    C. Sickle-cell anaemia
    D. Myelofibrosis

116. **Transient myeloproliferative disorder of the newborn is commonly seen in association with**
    A. Hurler syndrome
    B. Down's syndrome
    C. Ataxia telangiectasia
    D. Froehlich's syndrome

117. **Total serum LDH is not raised in**
    A. Stroke
    B. AMI
    C. Haemolysis
    D. Crush injury

118. **Sezary syndrome is**
    A. B-cell lymphoma
    B. Arsenical hyperkeratosis
    C. T-cell lymphoma
    D. A variety of alopecia mucinosa

119. **Histiocytosis X disease does not include**
    A. Hand-Schuller-Christian disease
    B. Niemann-Pick disease
    C. Letterer-Siwe disease
    D. Unifocal eosinophilic granuloma

120. **G6PD may reflect 'false normal' report in**
    A. Iron deficiency anaemia
    B. Hypoplastic anaemia
    C. Hairy cell leukaemia
    D. Shortly after haemolysis

Ans: 113-D 114-A 115-C 116-B 117-A 118-C 119-B 120-D

121. **Most sensitive and specific test for diagnosis of iron deficiency anaemia is**
   A. Serum ferritin level
   B. Percentage of transferrin saturation
   C. Serum transferrin receptor population
   D. Serum iron level

122. **Microcytic hypochromic anaemia is characteristic of**
   A. Persons who are true vegetarians
   B. Munchausen's syndrome
   C. Pseudohypoparathyroidism
   D. Patterson-Kelly syndrome

123. **Half-life of platelet is**
   A. 1–2 days
   B. 3–4 days
   C. 5–6 days
   D. 7–8 days

124. **Largest "organ system' in human body is**
   A. Blood
   B. Skin
   C. Endothelium
   D. GI tract

125. **Which of the following is not associated with microangiopathic blood picture**
   A. Thrombotic thrombocytopenic purpura
   B. Meningococcal septicaemia
   C. Severe burns
   D. Infectious mononucleosis (glandular fever)

126. **Macrocytosis of RBC is characteristic of all *except***
   A. Anaemia of myxoedema
   B. Methotrexate-induced
   C. Chronic alcoholism-induced liver disease
   D. Systemic lupus erythematosus

127. **Features of sickle-cell anaemia do not include**
   A. Nocturia
   B. Priapism
   C. Hypersplenism
   D. Leg ulcers

128. **Pancytopenia may develop from all *except***
   A. Haemosiderosis
   B. Paroxysmal nocturnal haemoglobinuria (PNH)
   C. Acute myeloid leukaemia (AML)
   D. Systemic lupus erythematosus

Ans: 121-A 122-D 123-B 124-C 125-D 126-D 127-C 128-A

129. Which of the following is associated with prolonged bleeding time

    A. Polycythaemia vera
    B. von Willebrand's disease
    C. Antiphospholipid syndrome
    D. Haemophilia

130. Peripheral blood picture is the most useful diagnostic aid in

    A. Non-Hodgkin's lymphoma   B. Multiple myeloma
    C. Myelodysplastic syndrome D. Chronic myeloid leukaemia

131. Gaisbock's syndrome is associated with

    A. Autoimmune haemolytic anaemia
    B. Paroxysmal nocturnal haemoglobinuria
    C. Stress erythrocytosis
    D. Idiopathic thrombocytopenic purpura

132. Which of the following is false in polycythaemia vera

    A. High erythropoietin level   B. Massive splenomegaly
    C. Hyperviscosity   D. Normal arterial saturation

133. Splenectomy is contraindicated in

    A. Pyruvate kinase deficiency
    B. Immune thrombocytopenic purpura
    C. Marrow failure
    D. Agnogenic myeloid metaplasia

134. Serum alkaline phosphatase level in multiple myeloma is usually

    A. Low   B. Normal
    C. Fluctuates   D. High

135. α-interferon is not beneficial in

    A. Hairy cell leukaemia
    B. Kaposi's sarcoma
    C. Chronic myeloid leukaemia
    D. Chronic granulomatous disease

136. Coagulation factor deficient in stored blood is

    A. VII   B. V
    C. IX   D. II

137. Punctate basophilia is seen in all *except*

    A. Megaloblastic anaemia   B. Thalassaemia
    C. Lead poisoning   D. Iron deficiency anaemia

Ans: 129-B 130-D 131-C 132-A 133-C 134-B 135-D 136-B 137-D

138. **Lifespan of platelets is**
   - A. 2–4 days
   - B. 5–7 days
   - C. 9–11 days
   - D. 13–15 days

139. **Half-life of albumin is**
   - A. 1–2 days
   - B. 10–14 days
   - C. 16-20 days
   - D. 20–26 days

140. **Burr-cells in the blood are seen in**
   - A. Cirrhosis of liver
   - B. Myxoedema
   - C. Haemolytic anaemia
   - D. Uraemia

141. **Which of the following factors is unstable in stored blood**
   - A. II
   - B. V
   - C. VII
   - D. X

142. **Megakaryocytosis in bone marrow is seen in all** *except*
   - A. Myeloid metaplasia
   - B. Polycythaemia vera
   - C. Chronic myeloid leukaemia
   - D. Idiopathic thrombocytopenic purpura

143. **Parahaemophilia is deficiency of factor**
   - A. IX
   - B. V
   - C. XI
   - D. von Willebrand's

144. **X-linked recessive inheritance is found in**
   - A. Red-green colour blindness
   - B. Blood group X (g)
   - C. Incontinentia pigmentii
   - D. Vitamin D resistant rickets

145. **Haemolysis in subjects with G6PD deficiency is reported with all** *except*
   - A. Chloramphenicol
   - B. Ciprofloxacin
   - C. Carbamazepine
   - D. Naphthalene (moth-balls)

146. **Thrombasthenia may be seen in all of the following** *except*
   - A. Diabetes mellitus
   - B. Paraproteinaemia
   - C. Myeloproliferative disorders
   - D. Uraemia

147. **Low-dose arsenic trioxide has recently been used in relapsed patients of**
   - A. Acute lymphoblastic leukaemia
   - B. Aplastic anaemia
   - C. Hairy cell leukaemia
   - D. Acute promyelocytic leukaemia

Ans: 138-C 139-D 140-D 141-B 142-C 143-B 144-A 145-C 146-A 147-D

8

Poisoning, Toxins and Environmental Hazards

1. **The cerebral syndrome after radiation does not include**
   - A. Vomiting
   - B. Convulsions
   - C. Blindness
   - D. Ataxia

2. **Which of the following is false in heat exhaustion**
   - A. Skin is cold and clammy
   - B. BP is low
   - C. Pulse pressure is elevated
   - D. Constricted pupils

3. **Which of the following is not a sign of atropinisation**
   - A. Dilated and reactive pupil
   - B. Rise of surface temperature
   - C. Dry mouth
   - D. Tachycardia

4. **In a G6PD-deficient subject, ingestion of which of the following may produce haemolysis**
   - A. Oxalic acid
   - B. Phenol
   - C. Salicylates
   - D. Naphthalene

5. **Which of the following is a recognised complication of methyl alcohol poisoning**
   - A. Blindness
   - B. Convulsions
   - C. Respiratory distress
   - D. Metabolic alkalosis

6. **All are modalities of treatment in carbon monoxide poisoning** *except*
   - A. Hyperbaric oxygen
   - B. Physostigmine
   - C. Artificial ventilation
   - D. Blood transfusion

7. **As a first line treatment, Elapidae group of snake bite should receive**
   - A. Neostigmine
   - B. Atropine
   - C. Polyvalent antivenin
   - D. Blood

8. **Sudden death as a result of severe electrical shock is commonly due to**
   - A. Circulatory collapse
   - B. Ventricular fibrillation
   - C. Hypovolaemic shock
   - D. Acute renal failure

Ans: 1-C 2-D 3-A 4-D 5-A 6-B 7-C 8-B

9. Intake of 8 g paracetamol as a single dose may produce
   A. Seizures
   B. Acute pancreatitis
   C. Cardiomyopathy
   D. Hepatic damage

10. Which of the following is not recognised as nicotinic effect of organophosphorus poisoning
    A. Fasciculation
    B. Flaccid paralysis
    C. Lacrimation
    D. Muscular twitching

11. IV ethanol therapy is treatment of choice in poisoning with
    A. Formaldehyde
    B. Methyl alcohol
    C. Glycols
    D. Isopropyl alcohol

12. Drowning features all of the following *except*
    A. 10–20% cases are 'dry' drowning
    B. Hypoxia is the most important problem in near drowning
    C. DIC may occur as a complication
    D. Metabolic alkalosis is an established complication

13. Drug of choice in paracetamol poisoning is
    A. Penicillamine
    B. Amyl nitrite
    C. N-acetylcystine
    D. Cholestyramine

14. Which of the following prevents cardiopulmonary complications in scorpion bite
    A. Inj. antivenin
    B. Local infiltration of lignocaine
    C. Corticosteroid
    D. Prazosin

15. Accidental hypothermia has been found in all *except*
    A. Cushing's syndrome
    B. Myxoedema
    C. Pituitary insufficiency
    D. Acute myocardial infarction

16. Endemic fluorosis is featured by all *except*
    A. Exostosis
    B. Kyphosis
    C. Chalky opacities on teeth
    D. Osteoporosis

17. Pink disease is heavy metal poisoning with
    A. Mercury
    B. Copper
    C. Arsenic
    D. Lead

18. Cigarette smoking is not a risk factor for development of
    A. Thromboangiitis obliterans
    B. Systemic hypertension
    C. Ischaemic heart disease
    D. Atherosclerosis

Ans: 9-D 10-C 11-B 12-D 13-C 14-D 15-A 16-D 17-A 18-B

19. Which of the following poisonings is not treated by penicillamine
    A. Copper   B. Antimony
    C. Lead   D. Mercury

20. Intermediate syndrome is seen in poisoning with
    A. Organophosphorus compound
    B. Benzodiazepines
    C. Mushrooms
    D. Cadmium

21. Rain-drop pigmentation is classical in poisoning with
    A. Antimony   B. Cadmium
    C. Arsenic   D. Copper

22. Basophilic stippling in RBC is found in poisoning with
    A. Mercury   B. Lead
    C. Gold   D. Cadmium

23. Victims of mushroom poisoning (*Amanita phalloides*) may die of
    A. Acute tubular necrosis
    B. Cardiac standstill
    C. Raised intracranial tension
    D. Acute hepatic necrosis

24. In mercury poisoning, death is usually due to
    A. Hepatocellular failure   B. Hypovolaemic shock
    C. Renal failure   D. Encephalopathy

25. Hyperkeratosis of palm and sole are seen in all *except*
    A. Tylosis   B. Arsenic poisoning
    C. Phrenoderma   D. Behcet's syndrome

26. In acute diazepam overdose, drug of choice for treatment is
    A. Acetylcysteine   B. Oximes
    C. Adrenaline   D. Flumazenil

27. Latic acidosis may develop from
    A. Glimepiride   B. Phenformin
    C. Repaglinide   D. Pioglitazone

28. Respiratory failure may complicate snake bite with
    A. Elapidae   B. Crotalidae
    C. Hydrophidae   D. Colubridae

Ans: 19-B 20-A 21-C 22-B 23-D 24-C 25-D 26-D 27-B 28-A

29. **Mees line is seen in poisoning with**
    - A. Lead
    - B. Arsenic
    - C. Copper
    - D. Bismuth

30. **Most of the absorbed lead in chronic poisoning is deposited in**
    - A. Hair
    - B. Nails
    - C. Bones
    - D. Liver

31. **The Prausnitz-Kustner reaction is related to**
    - A. Near-drowning
    - B. Necrotising vasculitis
    - C. Anaphylaxis
    - D. Atopy

32. **Amyl nitrite inhalation is useful in poisoning with**
    - A. Hydrocyanic acid
    - B. Organophosphorus compound
    - C. MAO-inhibitors
    - D. Methyl alcohol

33. **A bitter almond odour in breath may be detected in poisoning with**
    - A. Cadmium
    - B. Mercury
    - C. Hydrocyanic acid
    - D. Carbon monoxide

34. **Most important adverse effect of cisplatin is**
    - A. Cardiotoxicity
    - B. Pulmonary fibrosis
    - C. Neurotoxicity
    - D. Nephrotoxicity

35. **Which of the following drug-overdose (poisoning) is not treated by haemodialysis**
    - A. Benzodiazepines
    - B. Digoxin
    - C. Lithium
    - D. Barbiturate

36. **Dilated pupil occurs in poisoning with**
    - A. Neostigmine
    - B. Organophosphorus
    - C. Dhatura
    - D. Opium alkaloids

37. **Tricyclic antidepressants poisoning does not produce**
    - A. Dilated pupils
    - B. Salivation
    - C. Absent bowel sound
    - D. Cardiac dysrhythmias

38. **The temperature of burning cone of a cigarette is**
    - A. 400°C
    - B. 600°C
    - C. 900°C
    - D. 1400°C

Ans: 29-B 30-C 31-C 32-A 33-C 34-D 35-B 36-C 37-B 38-C

39. Blisters and bullae may develop over pressure points in poisoning with
   A. Carbon monoxide   B. Cyanide
   C. Hydrogen sulphide   C. Lithium

40. N-acetylcysteine may confer some protection against toxic effect of
   A. Nitrogen dioxide   B. Ammonia
   C. Phosgene   D. Carbon monoxide

41. Itai-itai (ouch-ouch) disease with renal tubular damage and osteomalacia is due to toxicity of
   A. Thallium   B. Vanadium
   C. Mercury   D. Cadmium

42. Regarding acid poisoning, which of the following is false
   A. Liquefactive necrosis of the GI tract mucosa
   B. Typically spares the oesophagus in majority
   C. Stridor may occur due to epiglottic oedema
   D. DIC may be a complication

43. 'Metal fume fever' is due to acute poisoning with
   A. Vanadium   B. Zinc oxide
   C. Manganese   D. Aluminium

44. Nitrazepam overdose is manifested as
   A. Paroxysmal atrial tachycardia   B. Mydriasis
   C. Hypothermia   D. Seizures

45. After intake of 40 tablets of aspirin, a person develops
   A. Hyperventilation   B. Unconsciousness
   C. Hyperglycaemia   D. Hypokalaemia

46. Phenothiazines may cause all of the following *except*
   A. Orthostatic hypotension B. Photosensitivity
   C. Extrapyramidal syndrome D. Impotence

47. Hyperostosis is seen in chemical poisoning with all *except*
   A. Arsenic   B. Fluoride
   C. Copper   D. Bismuth

48. Pin-point pupil is not a feature in poisoning with
   A. Dextroproxyphene
   B. Imipramine
   C. Organophosphorus compound
   D. Opiates

Ans: 39-A 40-C 41-D 42-A 43-B 44-C 45-A 46-D 47-C 48-B

49. Toxic level of lithium in serum is above
   A. 0.8 mEq/l   B. 1.1 mEq/l
   C. 1.3 mEq/l   D. 1.5 mEq/l

50. All of the following are true regarding benzodiazepines poisoning *except*
   A. Nystagmus   B. Bradypnoea
   C. Restlessness   D. Flumazenil used as antidote

51. Toxic level of phenytoin in serum is
   A. >10 µg/ml   B. >20 µg/ml
   C. > 30 µg/ml   D. >40 µg/ml

52. Chronic intoxication of which of the following metals give rise to gout
   A. Copper   B. Arsenic
   C. Mercury   D. Lead

53. Low uric acid level is characteristic of
   A. Early pregnancy   B. Psoriasis
   C. Down's syndrome   D. Lactic acidosis

54. Mode of action of pralidoxime is
   A. Sympathomimetic   B. Reactivate cholinesterase
   C. Inhibitis cholinesterase   D. Autonomic paralysis

55. Drug of choice in thallium poisoning is
   A. Cobalt edetate   B. Methylene blue
   C. Bromides   D. Prussian blue

56. Monge's disease is
   A. Chronic mountain sickness
   B. Chronic chromium deficiency
   C. Zinc toxicity
   D. Chronic selenium deficiency

57. Botulinum toxin A is not useful in
   A. Achalasia cardia   B. Trigeminal neuralgia
   C. Bell's palsy   D. Writer's cramp

58. Complaint of weakness as a result of long continued use of penicillamine is due to all *except*
   A. Myopathy   B. Severe arthralgia
   C. Anaemia   D. Myasthenia

Ans: 49-D 50-C 51-C 52-D 53-A 54-B 55-D 56-A 57-C 58-C

59. Which of the following is not a feature of chronic arsenicosis
    A. Guttate melanosis
    B. Non-cirrhotic hepatic fibrosis
    C. Beau's line in nails
    D. Basophilic stippling of erythrocytes

60. A patient of lathyrism should be differentiated from all of the following *except*
    A. Guillain-Barré syndrome
    B. HTLV myelopathy
    C. Primary lateral sclerosis
    D. Multiple sclerosis

61. Regarding investigations in fluorosis, which of the following is false
    A. High serum alkaline phosphatase
    B. Increased urinary hydroxyproline
    C. High serum calcium
    D. Elevated serum parathormone level

62. Haemodynamic, hormonal and metabolic effects of scorpion sting can be well antagonized by a single drug like
    A. Amiodarone
    B. Lignocaine
    C. Beta-blockers
    D. Prazosin

63. Which is not a recognized feature of 'disorder of high altitude'
    A. Retinopathy
    B. Pulmonary oedema
    C. Cerebral oedema
    D. Embolic episodes

Ans: 59-C 60-A 61-C 62-D 63-D

9

Infections and Infestations

1. **Ecthyma gangrenosum is produced by**
   - A. *Klebsiella*
   - B. *Serratia*
   - C. *Pseudomonas*
   - D. *Salmonella*

2. **Rifampicin is used in all *except***
   - A. Legionnaires' disease
   - B. Chemoprophylaxis of meningococcus meningitis
   - C. Leprosy
   - D. Bartonellosis

3. **Which of the following is not a live attenuated vaccine**
   - A. Rubella
   - B. Oral polio
   - C. Influenza
   - D. Mumps

4. **Most reliable clue to poor tissue perfusion in septic shock is**
   - A. High level of blood lactate
   - B. Hyponatraemia
   - C. Low level of HCO_3^-
   - D. Hypochloraemia

5. **Regarding scarlet fever, which statement is false**
   - A. Rash is mainly present in palms and soles
   - B. Raspberry tongue is seen
   - C. Previously Dick test was used for diagnosis
   - D. Confluent petechiae seen in this disease are known as Pastia's lines

6. **Commonest aetiologic agent of acute epiglottitis is**
   - A. *Streptococcus pneumoniae*
   - B. *Legionella pneumophilia*
   - C. *Staphylococcus aureus*
   - D. *Haemophilus influenzae*

7. **Majority of *Proteus* infection in humans is produced by**
   - A. *P. morganii*
   - B. *P. rettgeri*
   - C. *P. mirabilis*
   - D. *P. vulgaris*

Ans: 1-C 2-D 3-C 4-A 5-A 6-D 7-C

8. **Genital ulceration is caused by all** *except*

   A. Herpes simplex
   B. HIV
   C. *Treponema pallidum*
   D. *Haemophilus ducreyi*

9. **Agammaglobulinaemia patients are prone to be infected with**

   A. *Salmonella*
   B. *Staphylococcus aureus*
   C. *Streptococcus pneumoniae*
   D. *Pseudomonas*

10. **Fitz-Hugh-Curtis (perihepatitis) syndrome is caused by**

    A. *Meningococcus*
    B. *Gonococcus*
    C. *Pneumococcus*
    D. *Staphylococcus*

11. **The main pathogenic organism in non-gonococcal urethritis is**

    A. *Ureaplasma urealyticum*
    B. *Chalmydia trachomatis*
    C. Trichomoniasis
    D. Herpes simplex

12. **'Saint Anthony's fire' is**

    A. Bullous impetigo
    B. Ecthyma
    C. Facial haemangioma
    D. Erysipelas

13. **Shanghai fever or 13-day fever is caused by**

    A. *Haemophilus*
    B. *Pseudomonas*
    C. *Brucella*
    D. *Yersinia*

14. **In acute infection of melioidosis, the chief organ involved is**

    A. Brain
    B. Lung
    C. Liver
    D. Kidney

15. **Which of the following is not seen in typhoid state**

    A. Flapping tremor
    B. Coma vigil
    C. Subsultus tendinum
    D. Carphology

16. **Which of the following is false regarding Widal test**

    A. An agglutination reaction
    B. In vaccinated subjects, the O-titre disappears in time but H agglutinins present for years
    C. Titre of O-antigen above 1:640 is often very significant in enteric fever
    D. Antibiotic therapy may depress the agglutination titres

17. **All are indole +ve species of** *Proteus except*

    A. *P. mirabilis*
    B. *P. morganii*
    C. *P. vulgaris*
    D. *P. rettgeri*

Ans: 8-B 9-C 10-B 11-B 12-D 13-B 14-B 15-A 16-B 17-A

18. **Microbacterial flora of GI tract does not contain**
    A. *Bacteroides fragilis*
    B. *Pseudomonas*
    C. *Klebsiella ozaenae*
    D. *Clostridium perfringens*

19. **Which of the following features enteric fever in the first week**
    A. Continued type pyrexia
    B. Pea-soup diarrhoea
    C. Relative tachycardia
    D. Typhoid state

20. **Which is true in Widal test**
    A. Relapse bears relationship with agglutinin titre
    B. Agglutinin against flagellar antigen is most important
    C. Agglutinins begin to appear after 3rd day of infection
    D. Agglutinins reach a peak titre during the fifth or sixth week

21. **Which of the following is not characteristic of rose spots in typhoid fever**
    A. Appears during the early second week
    B. Do not blanch on pressure
    C. Erythematous macules
    D. They are bacterial emboli in skin capillaries

22. **Normal flora of mouth does not contain**
    A. *Actinomyces* species
    B. *Fusobacteria*
    C. Staphylococci
    D. *Escherichia* species

23. **Anti-pseudomonal activity is maximally present in**
    A. Ceftazidime
    B. Cefpodoxime proxetil
    C. Ceftriaxone
    D. Ceftizoxime

24. **Treatment of choice in chronic carrier of enteric fever is**
    A. Cholecystectomy
    B. Quinolones
    C. Ceftriaxone
    D. Furazolidone

25. **Malta fever is caused by**
    A. *Pasteurella tularensis*
    B. *Brucella abortus*
    C. *Haemophilus influenzae*
    D. *Pseudomonas mallei*

26. **Koch-Weeks bacillus is**
    A. *Haemophilus parainfluenzae*
    B. *Haemophilus aphrophilus*
    C. *Haemophilus ducreyi*
    D. *Haemophilus aegypticus*

Ans: 18-C 19-A 20-D 21-B 22-D 23-A 24-A 25-B 26-D

27. **All of the following are susceptible to have *Haemophilus* infections *except***

    A. G6PD deficiency
    B. Agammaglobulinaemia
    C. Splenectomised subject
    D. Sickle-cell disease

28. **Non-member of microbial flora of skin is**

    A. *Streptococcus faecalis*
    B. *Streptococcus epidermidis*
    C. *Erysipelothrix insidionna*
    D. *Streptococcus viridans*

29. **Which is false regarding brucellosis**

    A. Acquired through contact or ingestion of raw goat's milk
    B. *Brucella melitensis* is the most common type of infection
    C. CFT is more important in acute infection than that of agglutination reaction
    D. May present as pyrexia of unknown origin

30. **Which is not a recognised complication of acute shigellosis**

    A. Haemolytic-uraemic syndrome
    B. Reiter's syndrome
    C. Liver abscess
    D. Endotoxic shock

31. **Commonest cause of childhood otitis media is**

    A. *Haemophilus influenzae*
    B. *Pneumococcus*
    C. *Staphylococcus*
    D. *Pseudomonas*

32. **Which is not a complication of *Salmonella* species**

    A. Endocarditis
    B. Bronchiectasis
    C. Osteomyelitis
    D. Pyelonephritis

33. **Pseudobubo is caused by**

    A. *Haemophilus ducreyi*
    B. HIV
    C. Donovan body
    D. *Treponema pallidum*

34. **Woolsorter's disease is**

    A. Plague
    B. Legionnaires' disease
    C. Klebsiella-induced pneumonia
    D. Anthrax

35. **Botulism is manifested by all *except***

    A. Normal pupils
    B. Entirely normal sensory functions
    C. Increased protein in CSF
    D. Progressive descending muscle paralysis

Ans: 27-A 28-C 29-C 30-C 31-B 32-B 33-C 34-D 35-C

36. **Pontiac fever is due to**
    A. Serratia infection
    B. Acinetobacter infection
    C. Legionella infection
    D. Haemophilus infection

37. **Rat-bite fever is caused by the organism**
    A. *Spirillum minus*
    B. A gram-positive cocci
    C. *Yersinia multocida*
    D. *Treponema pertenue*

38. **Tuberculous focus in brain is known as**
    A. Rich's focus
    B. Wigard's focus
    C. Ashman's focus
    D. Simmon's focus

39. **The other name for Oroya fever is**
    A. Uveoparotid fever
    B. Rocky Mountain spotted fever
    C. Q fever
    D. Bartonellosis

40. **Which of the following is not a complication of Legionnaires' pneumonic illness**
    A. Disseminated intravascular coagulation
    B. Respiratory failure
    C. Encephalopathy
    D. Hypernatraemia

41. **Which of the neurological complications of diphtheria is last to appear**
    A. Loss of accommodation
    B. Peripheral neuropathy
    C. Bulbar palsy
    D. Bilateral Bell's palsy

42. **All of the following are seen in botulism *except***
    A. Increased salivation
    B. Ptosis
    C. Bulbar palsy
    D. Diplopia

43. *Cryptococcus neoformans* **is**
    A. A fungus
    B. Produces hepatosplenomegaly
    C. A higher bacteria
    D. Treated by IV lamivudine

44. **Jarisch-Herxheimer reaction may be seen in all *except***
    A. Syphilis after penicillin therapy
    B. Relapsing fever after receiving antimicrobials
    C. Enteric fever after ceftriaxone therapy
    D. Leprosy after dapsone therapy

Ans: 36-C 37-A 38-A 39-D 40-D 41-B 42-A 43-A 44-C

45. **Which of the following is not seen in secondary syphilis**
    A. Condylomata acuminatum
    B. Snail-track ulcers in mouth
    C. Generalised lymphadenopathy
    D. Skin rash

46. **All are stigma of congenital syphilis** *except*
    A. Mulberry molars
    B. Charcot joints
    C. Sabre tibia
    D. Interstitial keratitis

47. **Which of the following is false in Weil's disease**
    A. Leucopenia
    B. Conjunctival suffusion
    C. Azotaemia
    D. Meningism

48. **Thalidomide may be used in**
    A. Ulcerative colitis
    B. Kaposi's sarcoma
    C. Erythema nodosum leprosum
    D. Acute lung injury

49. **Cyclical periods of pyrexia alternating with apyrexia is found in all** *except*
    A. Relapsing fever
    B. Leprosy
    C. Hodgkin's disease
    D. Brucellosis

50. **The skin rash of secondary syphilis is**
    A. Itchy
    B. Asymmetrical
    C. Palms are not affected
    D. Pale red or pink in colour

51. **Which is the most sensitive test for syphilis**
    A. Wasserman test
    B. Rapid plasma reagin (RPR)
    C. VDRL
    D. Fluorescent treponemal antibody-absorption (FTA-ABS)

52. **Lymph node involvement in the usual site of disease is seen in infection by**
    A. *Mycobacterium avium-intracellulare*
    B. *Mycobacterium fortuitum*
    C. *Mycobacterium xenopi*
    D. *Mycobacterium scrofulaceum*

53. **Which valve is commonly involved in** *Coxiella burnetii* **(Q fever) endocarditis**
    A. Mitral
    B. Tricuspid
    C. Aortic
    D. Pulmonary

Ans: 45-A 46-B 47-A 48-C 49-B 50-D 51-D 52-D 53-C

54. **Which of the following is true in Kawasaki's disease**
    A. Common in middle age
    B. Pericardial invlovement is common
    C. High ASO titre
    D. Aneurysm of coronary arteries

55. **Weil-Felix reaction is negative in**
    A. Rocky Mountain spotted fever B. Rickettsial pox
    C. Epidemic typhus   D. Scrub typhus

56. **Which of the viral infections may be complicated by Reye's syndrome**
    A. Influenza   B. Hepatitis B
    C. Rubella   D. Coxsackie

57. **The cold agglutinin reaction is positive in**
    A. Endemic typhus   B. Sporotrichosis
    C. Relapsing fever   D. Mycoplasma infection

58. **Drug of choice in pneumonic legionellosis is**
    A. Rifampicin   B. Ceftizidime .
    C. Erythromycin   D. Co-amoxyclav

59. **Herpangina is due to infection caused by**
    A. Rubeola virus   B. Coxsackie A virus
    C. Adenovirus   D. Cytomegalovirus

60. **Vitamin K is synthesized in the gut by**
    A. *Bacteroides fragilis*   B. *Fusobacterium*
    C. *Bifidobacterium*   D. *Eubacterium*

61. **Which of the following is an RNA virus**
    A. Papovavirus   B. Herpesvirus
    C. Coronavirus   D. Adenovirus

62. **Q fever is transmitted to human by**
    A. Flea   B. Body louse
    C. Ticks   D. Mites

63. **Which of the following is not associated with measles**
    A. Transient loss of PPD (purified protein derivative)
    B. Remission of Hodgkin's disease
    C. Warthin-Finkeldey cells in hyperplastic lymphoid tissue
    D. Lighter maculopapular lesions than rubella

Ans: 54-D 55-B 56-A 57-D 58-C 59-B 60-A 61-C 62-C 63-D

64. **Faget's sign (relative bradycardia) is found in**
   A. Typhoid fever
   B. Yellow fever
   C. Acute rheumatic fever
   D. Brucellosis

65. **Cat-scratch disease is characterised by all *except***
   A. Regional lymphadenopathy
   B. Erythema nodosum
   C. Positive Hanger-Rose intradermal test
   D. Treated by antibiotic and corticosteroid

66. **Epstein-Barr virus is associated with all *except***
   A. Nasopharyngeal carcinoma
   B. Hairy cell leukaemia
   C. Burkitt's lymphoma
   D. Infectious mononucleosis

67. **Forchheimer's spots in soft palate are seen in**
   A. Rubella infection (German measles)
   B. Rubeola infection (measles)
   C. Yellow fever
   D. Dengue

68. **HSV-1 is associated with all *except***
   A. Genital vesicles
   B. Eczema herpeticum
   C. Acute gingivostomatitis
   D. Keratoconjunctivitis

69. **Presternal oedema is classically seen in**
   A. Measles
   B. Rabies
   C. Mumps
   D. Infectious mononulceosis

70. **Which is false in glandular fever (infectious mononucleosis)**
   A. Splenomegaly
   B. Ampicillin-induced skin rash
   C. Positive monospot test
   D. Acyclovir helps cure

71. **Bornholm's disease (pleurodynia) results from**
   A. Cytomegalovirus
   B. Coxsackie B virus
   C. Vaccinia virus
   D. Adenovirus

72. **Congenital rubella is not associated with**
   A. Corneal clouding
   B. Cardiac malformations
   C. Mental retardation
   D. Macrocephaly

Ans: 64-B 65-D 66-B 67-A 68-A 69-C 70-D 71-B 72-D

73. **Cerebral malaria is**
    A. Treated by oral quinine sulphate
    B. Often complicated by multi-organ failure
    C. Associated with signs of meningeal irritation
    D. IV dexamethasone reduces mortality rate

74. **Regarding primary amoebic meningoencephalitis, which is false**
    A. Almost invariably fatal
    B. Caused by *Naegleria fowleri*
    C. Dehydroemetine is drug of choice
    D. Acquired by swimming in fresh warm water

75. **'River blindness' is due to**
    A. Toxoplasmosis   B. Onchocerciasis
    C. Trichinosis   D. Cysticerosis

76. **Haemorrhagic fever may be produced by all *except***
    A. Chikungunya   B. Yellow fever
    C. Dengue   D. Colorado tick fever

77. **Which of the following is false in tropical splenomegaly syndrome**
    A. Very high level of serum IgG
    B. Sinusoidal lymphocytosis on liver biopsy
    C. High malarial antibody titre
    D. Associated with massive splenomegaly

78. **Drug of choice in *Pneumocystis carinii* pneumonia is**
    A. Pentamidine isethionate   B. Zidovudine
    C. Cefoperazone   D. Aztreonam

79. **Which of the following is not a recognised complication of infectious mono-nucleosis**
    A. Guillain-Barré syndrome
    B. Meningoencephalitis
    C. Myoclonus
    D. Transverse myelitis

80. **In hepatic amoebiasis**
    A. Left lobe is commonly affected
    B. Liver function tests (LFT) are of diagnostic value
    C. Jaundice is uncommon
    D. Serological tests are not helpful in diagnosis

Ans: 73-B 74-C 75-B 76-D 77-A 78-A 79-C 80-C

81. **Rectal biopsy is diagnostic in all of the following** *except*
    - A. Amoebiasis
    - B. Strongyloidosis
    - C. Amyloidosis
    - D. Schistosomiasis

82. **Which is false in acute acquired toxoplasmosis**
    - A. Absence of cerebral calcification
    - B. Severe than congenital form
    - C. Lymphadenopathy is the most common clinical manifestation
    - D. Ocular manifestation is very rare

83. **Herpes labialis is classically seen in**
    - A. Enteric fever
    - B. Lobar pneumonia
    - C. Kala-azar
    - D. Pulmonary tuberculosis

84. **Koplik's spot is diagnostic of**
    - A. Mumps
    - B. Enteric fever
    - C. Measles
    - D. Diphtheria

85. **Which is not a cause of aseptic fever**
    - A. SLE
    - B. Crush injury
    - C. AIDS
    - D. Pontine haemorrhage

86. **Romana's sign is classically found in infection by**
    - A. *Schistosoma mansoni*
    - B. *Trypanosoma cruzi*
    - C. *Pneumocystis carinii*
    - D. *Toxoplasma gondii*

87. **Which of the following is not a feature of familial mediterranean fever**
    - A. Autosomal dominant disorder
    - B. Abdominal pain occurs in majority
    - C. Amyloidosis is a recognised complication
    - D. Colchicine is the drug of choice for treatment

88. **Leonine-like face is seen in all** *except*
    - A. Amyloidosis
    - B. Carcinoid syndrome
    - C. Dermatomyositis
    - D. Lepromatous leprosy

89. **Which of the following is false in hydatid disease of liver**
    - A. Caused by larval stage of *Echinococcus granulosus*
    - B. Diagnostic aspiration may produce anaphylaxis
    - C. Casoni's test is positive in all
    - D. Albendazole therapy is most efficacious

Ans: 81-B 82-D 83-B 84-C 85-C 86-B 87-A 88-C 89-C

90. **Acute kala-azar is diagnosed by all of the following** *except*
    A. Complement fixation test
    B. Counterimmunoelectrophoresis
    C. Bone marrow aspiration for LD bodies
    D. Aldehyde test

91. **Cysticercosis is the larval stage of**
    A. *Taenia solium*
    B. *Hymenolepiasis nana*
    C. *Taenia saginata*
    D. *Ancylostoma duodenale*

92. **Which of the following does not produce hypothermia**
    A. Neuroleptic malignant syndrome
    B. Panhypopituitarism
    C. Peripheral circulatory failure
    D. Myxoedema coma

93. **False-positive serological test for syphilis is not given by**
    A. Leprosy
    B. Glandular fever
    C. Malaria
    D. Tuberculosis

94. **Frei test is diagnostic of**
    A. Histoplasmosis
    B. Lymphogranuloma venereum
    C. Cat-scratch disease
    D. Scrub typhus

95. **Suramin is the drug of choice in**
    A. Endemic typhus
    B. Schistosomiasis
    C. African trypanosomiasis
    D. Q fever

96. **Myiasis is caused by**
    A. Fungus
    B. Virus
    C. Larvae of flies
    D. Rickettsia

97. **Tularaemia may produce all the following manifestations** *except*
    A. Conjunctivitis
    B. Mental confusions
    C. Painful lymphadenopathy
    D. Circulatory failure

98. **The 'Rumpel-Leede phenomenon' is typical of**
    A. Rocky Mountain spotted fever
    B. Endemic typhus
    C. Rickettsial pox
    D. Epidemic typhus

Ans: 90-D 91-A 92-A 93-D 94-B 95-C 96-C 97-D 98-A

99. **Diphtheria may be associated with all** *except*
    A. Toxic neuritis
    B. Myocarditis
    C. Meningitis
    D. Bull-neck

100. **Rose spot, if present, is diagnostic of**
    A. Grandular fever
    B. Malta fever
    C. Scarlet fever
    D. Enteric fever

101. **Severe cases of lassa fever may be associated with all** *except*
    A. Respiratory failure
    B. Renal failure
    C. Circulatory failure
    D. Hepatic failure

102. **Ducrey's skin test diagnoses**
    A. Tularaemia
    B. Brucellosis
    C. Chancroid
    D. Histoplasmosis

103. **Which secondary neoplasm is not related to AIDS**
    A. Non-Hodgkin's lymphoma
    B. Primary lymphoma of brain
    C. Carcinoma of the cervix
    D. Kaposi's sarcoma

104. **In syphilis, primary chancre occurs in all the sites** *except*
    A. Within the anal mucosa in anal intercourse
    B. Vagina
    C. Within the urethra
    D. Cervix

105. **Herpes zoster most commonly affects**
    A. Anterior horn cells
    B. Posterior root ganglia
    C. Sympathetic ganglia
    D. White matter of brain

106. **Non-specific urethritis complicates as**
    A. Impotence
    B. Ankylosing spondylitis
    C. Reactive arthritis
    D. Carcinoma of the cervix

107. **Dapsone is used in the treatment of all** *except*
    A. Dermatitis herpetiformis
    B. Toxoplasmosis
    C. Leprosy
    D. Cryptosporidiasis

108. **All of the following are recognised causes of seizures in a patient of AIDS** *except*
    A. Glioma
    B. AIDS-dementia complex
    C. Cerebral toxoplasmosis
    D. Cryptococcal meningitis

Ans: 99-C 100-D 101-A 102-C 103-C 104-C 105-B 106-C 107-D 108-A

109. **Initial site for cryptococcal infection is**
    - A. Bone
    - B. Lungs
    - C. Skin
    - D. Meninges

110. **The recognised toxicity of zalcitabine is**
    - A. Interstitial nephritis
    - B. Pancreatitis
    - C. Swelling of salivary glands
    - D. Cardiomyopathy

111. **Which of the following is not a cysticidal drug in amoebiasis**
    - A. Tetracycline
    - B. Diloxanide furoate
    - C. Chloroquine
    - D. Paromomycin

112. **HTLV-2 may be associated with**
    - A. Hairy cell leukaemia
    - B. Tropical spastic paraplegia
    - C. Burkitt's lymphoma
    - D. Hodgkin's disease

113. **Non-specific urethritis is associated with all *except***
    - A. *Chlamydia trachomatis*
    - B. *Trichomonas vaginalis*
    - C. Herpes simplex
    - D. *Ureaplasma urealyticum*

114. **The drug of choice in gonorrhoea is**
    - A. Procaine penicillin
    - B. Benzathine penicillin
    - C. Benzyl penicillin
    - D. Phenoxymethyl penicillin

115. **Charcot's joint may be found in all *except***
    - A. Diabetes mellitus
    - B. Reiter's syndrome
    - C. Leprosy
    - D. Tabes dorsalis

116. **Commonest malignancy found in an AIDS patient is**
    - A. Leukaemia
    - B. Lymphoma
    - C. Kaposi's sarcoma
    - D. Mycosis fungoides

117. **Skin lesions in secondary syphilis may take any of the following forms *except***
    - A. Vesicular
    - B. Maculopapular
    - C. Follicular
    - D. Psorasiform

118. **Which of the following is not a neurological complication of measles**
    - A. Encephalitis
    - B. Transverse myelitis
    - C. Peripheral neuropathy
    - D. Subacute sclerosing panencephalitis

Ans: 109-B 110-B 111-A 112-A 113-B 114-A 115-B 116-C 117-A 118-C

119. **Complications of gonorrhoea do not include**
    A. Endocarditis
    B. Arthritis
    C. Epididymo-orchitis
    D. Urethro-enteric fistula

120. **Which of the following drug is not used in *Pneumocystis carinii* infection**
    A. Dapsone
    B. Pentamidine
    C. Corticosteroid
    D. Co-trimoxazole

121. **As a complication, lymphogranuloma venereum does not produce**
    A. Perirectal abscess
    B. Rectal stricture
    C. Septicaemia
    D. Extensive scarring

122. **Drug of choice in cysticercosis is**
    A. Suramin
    B. Albendazole
    C. Metrifonate
    D. Niclosamide

123. **The fourth-generation cephalosporin is**
    A. Cefepime
    B. Ceftibuten
    C. Cefuroxime axetil
    D. Cefamandole

124. **Terbinafine is an**
    A. Antiprotozoal agent
    B. Antiviral agent
    C. Antibacterial agent
    D. Antifungal agent

125. **Thalidomide may be used in all *except***
    A. HIV-associated aphthous ulcers
    B. Behcet's disease
    C. Reactive arthritis
    D. Pyoderma gangrenosum

126. **In an immunocompromised patient, cytomegalovirus commonly produces**
    A. Encephalitis
    B. Hepatitis
    C. Myelitis
    D. Retinitis

127. **Drug-induced cataract may develop from all *except***
    A. Ethambutol
    B. Busulphan
    C. Phenothiazines
    D. Corticosteroids

128. **In syphilis, the response to treatment is best monitored by**
    A. TPI
    B. FTA-ABS
    C. TPHA
    D. VDRL

Ans: 119-D 120-C 121-C 122-B 123-A 124-D 125-C 126-D 127-A 128-D

129. **AIDS-chorioretinitis is commonly due to infection by**
    A. *Toxoplasma gondii*   B. Cytomegalovirus
    C. *Candida albicans*   D. *Cryptococcus neoformans*

130. **Fluoroquinolones resistance in enteric fever is due to**
    A. Plasmid-mediated
    B. Interference with antibiotic transport into the cells
    C. Chromosomally-mediated
    D. Not definitly known

131. **Infectious mononucleosis-like syndrome may occur in**
    A. HIV infection   B. Typhus
    C. Kawasaki's disease   D. Scarlet fever

132. **'Rigor' is not characteristic of**
    A. Acute pyelonephritis   B. Acute cholangitis
    C. Acute rheumatic carditis   D. Acute thrombophlebitis

133. **Characteristics of brucellosis are all *except***
    A. Marked sweating   B. Leucopenia
    C. Spondylitis   D. Mental depression

134. **Acquired toxoplasmosis features**
    A. Anterior uveitis
    B. Neutrophilic leucocytosis
    C. Cervical lymphadenopathy
    D. Exudative pharyngitis

135. **Infectious mononucleosis-like syndrome may result from all *except***
    A. Adenovirus type B   B. Cytomegalovirus
    C. Epstein-Barr virus   D. *Toxoplasma gondii*

136. **Splenectomised patients are prone to be infected with all *except***
    A. *Haemophilus influenzae*   B. *Babesia*
    C. *Streptococcus pneumoniae* D. *Staphylococcus albus*

137. **Surface temperature 1–2° higher on paralysed side is known as**
    A. Macewen's sign   B. Victor H'orsely's sign
    C. Hamman's sign   D. Homan's sign

138. **Malignant otitis externa is commonly caused by**
    A. *Pseudomonas pyocyaneus*   B. *Staphylococcus*
    C. *Pneumococcus*   D. *Haemophilus influenzae*

Ans: 129-B 130-C 131-A 132-C 133-B 134-C 135-A 136-D 137-B 138-A

139. Helminthiasis causing persistent fever is
- A. Trichinosis
- B. *Taenia solium* infestation
- C. *Hymenolepiasis nana* infestation
- D. Trichuriasis

140. Which of the anti-retroviral drugs is a protease-inhibitor
- A. Stavudin
- B. Nevirapine
- C. Saquinavir
- D. Abacavir

141. Borrelia infection does not produce
- A. Lyme disease
- B. Tropical ulcer
- C. Yaws
- D. Relapsing fever

142. Epstein-Barr virus produces
- A. Cervical carcinoma
- B. Tropical spastic paraparesis
- C. Kaposi's sarcoma
- D. Nasopharyngeal carcinoma

143. Malignant otitis externa is common in
- A. Amyloidosis
- B. Lyme disease
- C. Diabetes mellitus
- D. Diphtheria

144. 'Croup' happens to occur due to affection by
- A. Parainfluenza virus
- B. *Haemophilus infleunzae*
- C. *Streptococcus pneumoniae*
- D. Herpes simplex virus

145. Commonest sexually transmitted disease (STD) is
- A. AIDS
- B. Non-gonococcal urethritis
- C. Gonorrhoea
- D. Genital warts

146. Haverhill fever is due to
- A. *Streptobacillus moniliformis*
- B. *Spirillum minus*
- C. *Pseudomonas aeruginosa*
- D. *Streptococcus pneumoniae*

147. Which is not HIV-related malignancy
- A. Non-Hodgkin's lymphoma
- B. Sinus histocytosis
- C. Invasive cervical carcinoma
- D. Primary lymphoma of brain

148. Which is false in *Pneumocystis carinii* pneumonia in AIDS
- A. Most common opportunistic infection
- B. Diffuse perihilar infiltrates in chest X-ray
- C. Pleural effusions are common
- D. Aerosolized pentamidine therapy may produce pneumothorax

Ans: 139-A 140-C 141-C 142-D 143-C 144-A 145-B 146-A 147-B 148-C

149. **Hutchinson's triad in congenital syphilis does not include**
    A. Interstitial keratitis
    B. Rhagades
    C. Peg-shaped upper central incisors
    D. Nerve deafness

150. **All of the following produce viral haemorrhagic fever** *except*
    A. Lassa fever virus
    B. Norwalk virus
    C. Ebola virus
    D. Congo-Crimean haemorrhagic fever virus

151. *Isospora belli* **infection is treated by**
    A. Cotrimoxazole   B. Amoxycillin
    C. Chloramphenicol   D. Streptomycin

152. **Oedema of the face and periorbital tissue are found in**
    A. Toxocariasis   B. Strongyloidosis
    C. Trichuriasis   D. Trichinosis

153. **Which of the following is not regarded as a biological weapon**
    A. Chickenpox   B. Plague
    C. Botulism   D. Tularaemia

Ans: 149-B 150-B 151-A 152-D 153-A

1. Which of the following statement is false regarding SIADH
   A. Plasma osmolality is < 270 mOsm/kg
   B. Complains of weakness, lethargy and weight gain
   C. Urine is almost always hypertonic to plasma
   D. Presence of pitting oedema

2. Hyponatraemia is manifested by all *except*
   A. Muscular weakness   B. Paralytic ileus
   C. Myoclonic jerks   D. Confusion

3. All are established causes of SIADH *except*
   A. Meningitis   B. Hyperthyroidism
   C. Oat-cell carcinoma of lung   D. Acute intermittent porphyria

4. Kussmaul's respiration is characteristic of
   A. Metabolic alkalosis   B. Respiratory acidosis
   C. Metabolic acidosis   D. Respiratory alkalosis

5. Causes of hyponatraemia with normal extracellular fluid (ECF) are all *except*
   A. Nephrotic syndrome   B. Diabetic ketoacidosis
   C. Hypothyroidism   D. Use of diuretics

6. Volume depletion (combined Na^+ and water depletion) does not occur in
   A. Cirrhosis of liver   B. Peritonitis
   C. Chronic renal failure   D. Adrenal insufficiency

7. 'Skin turgor' is best examined
   A. Over the abdominal parities
   B. Over the dorsum of hand
   C. Over the sternum
   D. Over the cheeks

Ans: 1-D 2-B 3-B 4-C 5-B 6-A 7-C

8. **All of the following produce hyponatraemia** *except*
   A. Prolonged use of frusemide
   B. SIADH
   C. Ulcerative colitis
   D. Diabetic ketoacidosis

9. **Polyuria, polydipsia associated with nocturia is not a feature of**
   A. Hypokalaemia
   B. Hyperparathyroidism
   C. CCF with diuretic therapy
   D. Hypermagnesaemia

10 **All are causes of 'sick-cell syndrome'** *except*
   A. Congestive cardiac failure
   B. Pulmonary tuberculosis
   C. Pericardial effusion
   D. Cirrhosis of liver

11. **Maximally dilute urine in a hyponatraemic patient suggests**
   A. Psychogenic polydipsia
   B. Adrenal failure
   C. Diabetic ketoacidosis
   D. SIADH

12. **Which of the following is not associated with hypokalaemia**
   A. Frusemide
   B. Triamterene
   C. Chlorthalidone
   D. Indapamide

13. **All of the following produce hypernatraemia** *except*
   A. Adults on high protein-calorie nasogastric feeding
   B. Diabetes insipidus
   C. Hypoaldosteronism
   D. Hyperosmolar non-ketotic diabetic coma

14. **Hypokalaemia is not produced by**
   A. Villous adenoma of large bowel
   B. Primary aldosteronism
   C. Ureterosigmoidostomy
   D. Metabolic acidosis

15. **After rapid correction of hyponatraemia in a patient, quadruparesis develops as a result of**
   A. Guillain-Barré syndrome
   B. Central pontine myelinolysis
   C. Periodic paralysis
   D. Acute transverse myelitis

16. **Hypokalaemia is not associated with**
   A. U-wave in ECG
   B. Decreased ankle jerk
   C. Oliguria
   D. Paralytic ileus

Ans: 8-C 9-D 10-C 11-A 12-B 13-C 14-D 15-B 16-C

17. **The normal serum potassium level is**
    A. 2.1–3.6 mEq/l
    B. 2.9–4.2 mEq/l
    C. 3.5–5.0 mEq/l
    D. 4.7–6.6 mEq/l

18. **Hypoprothrombinaemia features**
    A. Vitamin K deficiency
    B. Low platelet count
    C. Allergic purpura
    D. Increased capillary fragility

19. **Fanconi's syndrome is associated with all *except***
    A. Hypophosphataemia
    B. Hypokalaemia
    C. Hypouricaemia
    D. Hypocalciuria

20. **Hypokalaemia enhances the cardiac toxicity of**
    A. Amiodarone
    B. Propranolol
    C. Adenosine
    D. Digoxin

21. **Night blindness may develop from all *except***
    A. Retinitis pigmentosa
    B. Marasmus
    C. Hypovitaminosis A
    D. Zinc deficiency

22. **Metabolic alkalosis is associated with all the following *except***
    A. Severe vomiting
    B. Hypokalaemia
    C. Bartter's syndrome
    D. Methanol poisoning

23. **All of the following may be associated with carotinaemia *except***
    A. Anorexia nervosa
    B. Hypovitaminosis A
    C. Castrated male
    D. Myxoedema

24. **Which is not an aetiology of metabolic acidosis with normal anion gap**
    A. Hypoaldosteronism
    B. Diabetic ketoacidosis
    C. Diarrhoea
    D. Renal tubular acidosis

25. **Acute hyperkalaemia is treated by all *except***
    A. IV 10% calcium gluconate
    B. Glucose-insulin infusion
    C. IV frusemide
    D. Sodium polystyrene sulfonate retention enema

26. **Normal anion gap is**
    A. 2–4 mmol/l
    B. 4–8 mmol/l
    C. 8–16 mmol/l
    D. 16–24 mmol/l

Ans: 17-C 18-A 19-D 20-D 21-B 22-D 23-B 24-B 25-C 26-C

27. **Pseudohyperkalaemia results from all of the following *except***

    A. Leucocytosis
    B. Crush injury
    C. In vitro haemolysis
    D. Poor venepuncture technique

28. **Metabolic acidosis is not featured by**

    A. Hypoventilation
    B. Lassitude
    C. Vascular collapse
    D. Stupor

29. **The EGG feature of hyperkalaemia does not include**

    A. QT prolongation
    B. Tall T-wave
    C. Wide QRS complex
    D. Diminution of P-wave amplitude

30. **Which of the following is not a feature of metabolic acidosis**

    A. Reduced serum HCO_3^- concentration
    B. Reuced plasma H^+
    C. Elevated serum urea
    D. Reduced CO_2-combining power

31. **Respiratory alkalosis is not characterised by**

    A. Raised $Paco_2$
    B. Reduced H^+ concentration
    C. Reduced level of HCO_3^-
    D. Raised serum lactate and pyruvate

32. **All of the following are unmeasured anions (i.e. responsible for anion gap) *except***

    A. Sulphate
    B. Inorganic phosphates
    C. Polyanionic plasma proteins
    D. Chloride

33. **Respiratory acidosis is associated with all *except***

    A. Emphysema
    B. Salicylate intoxication
    C. Myasthenia gravis
    D. Cardiac arrest

34. **Which is not a feature of phenylketonuria**

    A. Mental retardation
    B. Corneal opacity
    C. Hypopigmentation
    D. Mousy odour of urine

35. **Which of the following is a feature of respiratory alkalosis**

    A. Asterixis
    B. Papilloedema
    C. Water-hammer pulse
    D. Tetany

36. **The clinical hallmark of homocystinuria is**

    A. Osteoporosis
    B. Mental retardation
    C. Dislocation of lens
    D. Thrombotic vascular disease

Ans: 27-B 28-A 29-A 30-B 31-A 32-D 33-B 34-B 35-D 36-C

37. Rothera's test is positive with all of the following ingredient *except*
    A. β-hydroxybutyric acid
    B. Acetone
    C. Drug treatment with salicylates
    D. Acetoacetic acid

38. 'Sweaty feet' odour is found in
    A. Argininaemia   B. Glutaric aciduria
    C. Hypervalinaemia   D. Isovaleric acidaemia

39. Starvation is thought to be life-threatening, when the body weight falls below
    A. 40% of normal   B. 50% of normal
    C. 60% of normal   D. 70% of normal

40. Which of the following is not elevated in serum in maple syrup urine disease
    A. Valine   B. Isoleucine
    C. Ornithine   D. Leucine

41. Lesch-Nyhan syndrome is characterised by all *except*
    A. Intracerebral calcification   B. Self-mutilation
    C. Choreoathetosis   D. Hyperuricaemia

42. Band keratopathy is found in all *except*
    A. Copper deposition in Wilson's disease
    B. Chloroquine crystals in treating DLE
    C. Iron deposition in haemochromatosis
    D. Cystine crystals in cystinosis

43. Acute gouty arthritis should be treated by
    A. Allopurinol   B. Probenecid
    C. Benzbromarone   D. Naproxen

44. Which has the highest percentage of involvement in haemo-chromatosis
    A. Splenomegaly
    B. Skin pigmentation
    C. Diabetes mellitus
    D. Cardiac involvement

45. Pellagra-like clinical syndrome is found in
    A. Histidinuria   B. Hartnup disease
    C. Cystinosis   D. Iminoglycinuria

Ans: 37-A 38-D 39-D 40-C 41-A 42-C 43-D 44-B 45-B

46. **Hypochromic anaemia with megaloblastic changes in bone marrow is seen in**
   A. Galactosaemia
   B. Abetalipoproteinaemia
   C. Gaucher's disease
   D. Hereditary orotic aciduria

47. **In cystinuria, which of the amino acids is not excreted in urine**
   A. Ornithine
   B. Cysteine
   C. Arginine
   D. Cystine

48. **All of the following may lead to hyperuricaemia *except***
   A. Thiazide diuretics
   B. High doses of aspirin
   C. Nicotinic acid
   D. Pyrazinamide

49. **Which is false in alcaptonuria (ochronosis)**
   A. X-ray of lumbar spine is virtually pathognomonic
   B. Pigmentation of skin
   C. Urine turns black upon alkalinization
   D. Photophobia

50. **All are the indications of treating asymptomatic hyperuricaemia *except***
   A. Patient becomes symptomatic
   B. Has a strong family H/O gout or nephrolithiasis
   C. 24-hrs urinary uric acid excretion >1100 mg
   D. Associated with hypertension and diabetes mellitus

51. **Increased urinary aminolevulinic acid and porphobilinogen are found in all *except***
   A. Infectious mononucleosis
   B. Lead poisoning
   C. Amyloidosis
   D. Acute intermittent porphyria

52. **von Gierke's disease results from deficiency of**
   A. Muscle phosphorylase
   B. Glycogen synthetase
   C. Glucose-6-phosphatase
   D. Liver phosphorylase kinase

53. **Which is not a feature of acute intermittent porphyria**
   A. Psychiatric disturbances
   B. Pain abdomen
   C. Peripheral neuropathy
   D. Diarrhoea

54. **Hereditary fructose intolerance presents with all *except***
   A. Postprandial hypoglycaemia
   B. Lactic acidosis
   C. Renal stones
   D. Dental caries

Ans: 46-D 47-B 48-B 49-D 50-D 51-C 52-C 53-D 54-D

55. **Which is considered to be a safe drug in porphyria**
    A. Chlorpromazine
    B. Barbiturates
    C. Oral contraceptive pills
    D. Chlorpropamide

56. **Galactosaemia does not feature**
    A. Cataract
    B. Seizures
    C. Intellectual impairment
    D. Development of cirrhosis of liver

57. **Type I glycogenosis (von Gierke's disease) is not associated with**
    A. Myoglobinuria
    B. Lipaemia retinalis
    C. Macroglossia
    D. Hypoglycaemia

58. **Point out the false one regarding familial lipoprotein lipase deficiency**
    A. Lipaemia retinalis
    B. Abdominal pain due to pancreatitis
    C. Accelerated atherosclerosis
    D. Eruptive xanthoma

59. **Probably the commonest form of glycogen storage disorder is**
    A. Type I glycogenosis
    B. Type III glycogenosis
    C. Type V glycogenosis
    D. Type VI glycogenosis

60. **Familial dysbetalipoproteinaemia (type 3 hyperlipoproteinaemia) is manifested by all *except***
    A. Fluminant atherosclerosis
    B. Palmar xanthoma
    C. Results from accumulation of remnant-like particles derived from VLDL
    D. Manifested before the age of 20

61. **Gaucher's disease is featured by all *except***
    A. Most commonly encountered lysosomal storage disorder
    B. Bone pain
    C. High serum alkaline phosphatase
    D. Hepatosplenomegaly

62. **Weber-Christian disease does not include**
    A. Panniculitis
    B. Evidence of pancreatic disease
    C. Erythema marginatum
    D. Vasculitis

Ans: 55-A 56-B 57-A 58-C 59-B 60-D 61-C 62-C

63. **Secondary hyperlipoproteinaemia is associated with all** *except*
   A. Acute alcoholism
   B. Diabetes mellitus
   C. Use of oral contraceptives
   D. Addison's disease

64. **Tay-Sachs gangliosidosis is characterised by all** *except*
   A. Vascular thrombosis
   B. Macroencephaly
   C. Ocular cherry-red spots
   D. Hyperacusis

65. **Tangier's disease is manifested by**
   A. Premature atherosclerosis
   B. Pigmentation of skin
   C. Low serum cholesterol level
   D. Haemolysis

66. **Hurler disease has all the following features** *except*
   A. Accumulation of heparan and dermatan sulphate
   B. Absence of corneal clouding
   C. Gibbus
   D. Beaking of the lumbar vertebrae

67. **Abetalipoproteinaemia is not characterised by**
   A. Ataxia
   B. Eruptive xanthoma
   C. Acanthocytosis
   D. Retinitis pigmentosa

68. **Fabry's disease does not include**
   A. Autosomal recessive inheritance
   B. Corneal dystrophy
   C. Cataract
   D. Deficiency of α-galactosidase

69. **Familial hypercholesterolaemia is characterised by all** *except*
   A. Obesity
   B. Xanthelasma
   C. Tendon xanthoma
   D. Arucus corneae

70. **Niemann-Pick disease is manifested by all** *except*
   A. Retinal cherry-red spots
   B. Elevated serum lipids level
   C. Results from deficiency of sphingomyelinase
   D. May be a part of 'sea blue histiocyte syndrome'

71. **Loose-jointedness occurs in all of the following** *except*
   A. Marfan's syndrome
   B. Ehlers-Danlos syndrome
   C. Osteogenesis imperfecta
   D. Pseudoxanthoma elasticum

Ans: 63-D 64-A 65-C 66-B 67-B 68-A 69-A 70-B 71-D

72. Osteogenesis imperfecta is manifested by all *except*

 A. Blue sclera
 B. Malar flush
 C. Recurrent fractures in long bones
 D. 'Wormian bones' in the skull

73. Hypomagnesaemia is associated with all *except*

 A. Hypercalcaemia
 B. Use of loop diuretics
 C. Acute pancreatitis
 D. Chronic renal failure

74. The most frequent CVS finding in Noonan syndrome is

 A. Pulmonary stenosis
 B. Coarctation of aorta
 C. Aortic stenosis
 D. Mitral valve prolapse

75. Marfan's syndrome is not featured by

 A. Metacarpal index >8.4
 B. Dolicocephaly
 C. Arachnodactyly
 D. Upper segment > lower segment of body

76. The best natural source of iodine is

 A. Meat
 B. Milk
 C. Vegetables
 D. Seafoods

77. Angioid streaks in the retina are seen in all *except*

 A. Paget's disease
 B. Hypophosphataemia
 C. Sickle cell anaemia
 D. Pseudoxanthoma elasticum

78. Laurence-Moon-Biedl syndrome is associated with

 A. Arachnodactyly
 B. Mitral valve prolapse
 C. Retinitis pigmentosa
 D. Slender body habitus

79. All of the following statements are true regarding Ehlers-Danlos syndrome *except*

 A. Pes cavus
 B. Type IV is the most dangerous type
 C. Hyperextensible skin
 D. Association with mitral valve prolapse

80. Antimongoloid slant of the eyes is not seen in

 A. Noonan syndrome
 B. Cri-du-chat syndrome
 C. Down's syndrome
 D. Treacher Collins syndrome

Ans: 72-B 73-D 74-A 75-D 76-D 77-B 78-C 79-A 80-C

81. **Obesity is not associated with**
    A. Hypogonadisn
    B. Hypopituitarism
    C. Hypocortisolism
    D. Hypothyroidism

82. **The most important diagnostic aid in rickets is**
    A. Low serum phosphate level
    B. High serum alkaline phosphatase level
    C. Low serum calcium level
    D. Normal serum urea and creatinine levels

83. **Vitamin D is maximally present in**
    A. Fatty fish
    B. Butter
    C. Milk
    D. Eggs

84. **'Keshan disease' is due to deficiency of**
    A. Manganese
    B. Cobalt
    C. Zinc
    D. Selenium

85. **Hyperphosphataemia is not associated with**
    A. Acute haemolysis
    B. Diabetic ketoacidosis
    C. Acute renal failure
    D. Rhabdomyolysis

86. **Menkes' kinky hair disease results from deficiency of**
    A. Copper
    B. Iron
    C. Fluoride
    D. Vanadium

87. **All are consequences of phosphate depletion *except***
    A. Cardiac arrhythmias
    B. Respiratory muscle weakness
    C. Hypocalciuria
    D. Neuroencephalopathy

88. **Zinc deficiency may lead to all *except***
    A. Gonadal atrophy
    B. Dermatitis
    C. Muscular weakness
    D. Diarrhoea

89. **Primary amyloidosis does not involve**
    A. Heart
    B. Spleen
    C. Kidney
    D. Brain

90. **Hypervitaminosis A does not manifest as**
    A. Cracked lips
    B. Begin intracranial hypertension
    C. Vomiting
    D. Phrenoderma

Ans: 81-C 82-B 83-A 84-D 85-B 86-A 87-C 88-C 89-D 90-D

91. **Amyloidosis may develop from all of the following** *except*

    A. Multiple myeloma
    B. Emphysema
    C. Leprosy
    D. Rheumatoid arthritis

92. **Sabre tibia is seen in**

    A. Thalassaemia major
    B. Achondroplasia
    C. Congenital syphilis
    D. Down's syndrome

93. **Pyridoxine (vit B₆) is used in all of the following** *except*

    A. Pregnancy-induced vomiting
    B. Sideroblastic anaemia
    C. Along with INH therapy
    D. Thalassaemia major

94. **Rickets is not manifested by**

    A. Sweating in forehead
    B. Flabby muscles
    C. Pectus excavatum
    D. Distended abdomen

95. **Hormone replacement therapy (HRT) in psotmenopausal women has all the potential risks** *except*

    A. Endometrial carcinoma
    B. Venous thromboembolism
    C. Ischaemic heart disease
    D. Breast carcinoma

96. **Osteoporosis results from**

    A. Hypoparathyroidism
    B. Late menopause
    C. Hypothyroidism
    D. Low body weight

97. **BMI (body mass index) range for simple obesity is**

    A. 18.5–24.9
    B. 25.0–29.9
    C. 30.0–39.9
    D. ≥40

98. **Riboflavin deficiency does not give rise to**

    A. Peripheral neuropathy
    B. Nasolabial seborrhoea
    C. Angular stomatitis
    D. Magenta-coloured tongue

99. **Which is not beneficial in the treatment of osteoporosis**

    A. Etidronate
    B. Sodium fluoride
    C. Corticosteroid
    D. Calcitriol

100. **Cheilosis may result from deficiency of all** *except*

    A. Iron
    B. Vitamin B₁₂
    C. Nicotinic acid
    D. Riboflavin

Ans: 91-B 92-C 93-D 94-C 95-C 96-D 97-C 98-A 99-C 100-B

101. All are true regarding osteoporosis *except*
    A. Bending of long bones
    B. Vertebral collapse
    C. Exaggeration of thoracic kyphosis
    D. Shortened trunk

102. Richest source of vitamin B_{12} is
    A. Green leafy vegetables   B. Meat and dairy products
    C. Fruits   D. Seafish

103. Normal serum value of calcium is
    A. 7–9 mg/dl   B. 8–9.5 mg/dl
    C. 9–11 mg/dl   D. 10.5–12.5 mg/dl

104. Protein-energy malnutrition is characterised by
    A. Sexual precocity
    B. Reduced by weight for age
    C. Pot-bellied abdomen with umbilical hernia
    D. Craniotabes

105. Which of the following is a single gene disorder
    A. Systemic hypertension   B. von Gierke's disease
    C. Retinoblastoma   D. Diabetes mellitus

106. Looser's zone in osteomalacia is seen in all of the following sites *except*
    A. Axillary border of scapula   B. Pubic rami
    C. Medial cortex of upper femur   D. Skull

107. Which of the following gives the surest test for diagnosis of gout
    A. Serum uric acid >13 mg/dl
    B. Classical punched-out lesion in X-ray
    C. Negative birefringent monosodium urate crystals on sinovial fluid examination
    D. 24-hrs urinary uric acid excretion > 1300 mg

108. Which is not characteristic of marasmus
    A. Marked wasting
    B. Irritable child
    C. Absence of hepatosplenomegaly
    D. Oedema

109. Diminished renal excretion of uric acid is seen in all *except*
    A. Severe exfoliative psoriasis   B. Myxoedema
    C. Lead poisoning   D. Mongolism

Ans: 101-A 102-B 103-C 104-B 105-C 106-D 107-C 108-D 109-A

110. Lactic acidosis results from all *except*

   A. Carbon monoxide poisoning   B. Chronic renal failure
   C. Diabetes mellitus   D. Biguanides-induced

111. Which is not an anti-obesity drug

   A. Sibutramine   B. Amitriptyline
   C. Orlistat   D. Fenfluramine

112. Cupping, widening and fraying of metaphyseal long bones are observed in all *except*

   A. Hypophosphatasia   B. Rickets
   C. Scurvy   D. Metaphyseal dysostosis

113. Calcification of intervertebral disc is characteristic of

   A. Chondrocalcinosis   B. Hypoparathyroidism
   C. Vitamin D toxicity   D. Ochronosis

114. Phagocytic cells with accumulation of sphingomyelin are found in

   A. Gaucher's disease   B. Fabry disease
   C. Neimann-Pick disease   D. Hunter syndrome

115. Night blindness may be due to all of the following *except*

   A. Cone dystrophy   B. Xeroderma pigmentosum
   C. Retinitis pigmentosa   D. Zinc-deficiency states

116. Serum homocysteine level may be elevated in all *except*

   A. Hypothyroidism   B. Chronic renal failure
   C. Psoriasis   D. COPD

117. Serum homocysteine lowering therapy is given by supplementation with

   A. Vitamin A and C   B. Folate, vitamin B_6 and B_{12}
   C. Riboflavin and nicotinic acid D. Biotin, vitamin C and B_6

118. Which is not an exogenous antioxidant

   A. α-tocopherol   B. Thiamine hydrochloride
   C. β-carotene   D. Ascorbic acid

119. Which is not having an autosomal dominant inheritance

   A. Glucose-6-phosphate dehydrogenase deficiency
   B. Huntington's chorea
   C. Neurofibromatosis
   D. Adult polycystic kidney

Ans: 110-B 111-B 112-C 113-D 114-C 115-A 116-D 117-B 118-B 119-A

120. **Hyperuricaemia is not associated with**
    A. Phosphoribosyl pyrophosphate synthetase overactivity
    B. Inhibition of xanthine oxidase
    C. Hypoxanthaine-guanine-phosphoribosyl transferase (HGPRT) deficiency
    D. Glucose-6-phosphatase deficiency

121. **Hypoglycaemia may result from all *except***
    A. Pentamidine   B. Octreotide
    C. Diazoxide   D. Quinine

122. **Plasma phosphate level is normal in**
    A. Renal osteodystrophy   B. Acromegaly
    C. Paget's disease   D. Rickets

123. **A high bicarbonate level is unusual in**
    A. Chronic cor pulmonale   B. Chronic renal failure
    C. Severe vomiting   D. Hypokalaemia

124. **Hyponatraemia is seen in**
    A. Hyperlipidaemia   C. Bronchogenic carcinoma
    C. Myxoedema coma   D. Cushing's syndrome

125. **Which of the following is not used to treat obesity**
    A. Phentolamine
    B. Recombinant human leptin
    C. Sibutramine
    D. Fenfluramine

126. **Pseudohyperkalaemia is noted in all *except***
    A. Marked leuocytosis   B. Use of tourniquet
    C. Acidosis   D. Thrombocytosis

127. **Which is an incompatible combination**
    A. Vomiting: Metabolic alkalosis
    B. Acute pulmonary oedema: Respiratory acidosis
    C. Diarrhoea: Metabolic acidosis
    D. Salicylate overdose: Respiratory alkalosis

128. **Metabolic acidosis with high anion gap is seen in all *except***
    A. Lactic acidosis
    B. Acute renal failure
    C. Ketoacidosis
    D. Ammonium chloride poisoning

Ans: 120-B 121-C 122-C 123-B 124-D 125-A 126-C 127-B 128-D

129. **In a critically ill patient, the most common acid-base disturbance is**
    A. Respiratory alkalosis
    B. Metabolic acidosis
    C. Respiratory acidosis
    D. Metabolic alkalosis

130. **Regarding pseudoxanthoma elasticum, which is false**
    A. Plucked chicken skin appearance
    B. CVA is the commonest mode of death
    C. Neck and axilla are commonly involved
    D. Long-term use of D-penicillamine may produce such skin lesion

131. **Lardaceous spleen is pathognomonic of**
    A. Chronic hepatitis
    B. Brucellosis
    C. Diffuse amyloidosis
    D. Sarcoidosis

132. **Pellagra may be manifested in all *except***
    A. Carcinoid syndrome
    B. Hartnup disease
    C. INH therapy
    D. Porphyria

133. **Vitamin C toxicity may result in**
    A. High uric acid
    B. Oxalate stones in kidney
    C. Loss of libido
    D. Sideroblastic anaemia

134. **Prognathism may be seen in**
    A. Noonan's syndrome
    B. Nemaline myopathy
    C. Turner's syndrome
    D. Marfan's syndrome

135. **GLUT-3 is most commonly seen in**
    A. Hepatocytes
    B. Pancreatic β-cells
    C. Adipocytes
    D. Brain

136. **Which is not included in 'lysosomal storage disorders'**
    A. Gaucher's disease
    B. Fabry's disease
    C. von Gierke's disease
    D. Niemann-Pick disease

137. **HDL can be significantly increased by**
    A. Lovastatin
    B. Nicotinic acid
    C. Clofibrate
    D. Gemfibrozil

Ans: 129-A 130-B 131-C 132-D 133-B 134-B 135-D 136-C 137-B

138. Which is included within definitive criteria of syndrome X
     A. Microalbuminuria
     B. ↑ C-reactive protein
     C. ↑ Homocysteine
     D. Type I diabetes mellitus

139. Guthrie's test is diagnostic of
     A. Homocystinuria
     B. Phenylketonuria
     C. Cystinosis
     D. Hartnup disease

140. Increased serum alkaline phosphatase is not characteristic of
     A. Osteoporosis
     B. Sarcoidosis
     C. Pregnancy
     D. Osteomalacia

141. Most characteristic feature of biotin deficiency is
     A. Anaemia
     B. Diarrhoea
     C. Perioral dermatitis
     D. Vascularisation of cornea

142. Which is not seen in hereditary orotic aciduria
     A. Hypochromic megaloblastic anaemia
     B. Hyperuicaemia
     C. Growth retardation
     D. Dietary supplement by uridine corrects anaemia

143. Regarding role of diet in treatment of hyperuricaemia, which of the following is false
     A. Dairy products reduce serum uric acid
     B. Sea food elevates serum uric acid
     C. Fructose in ice cream reduces serum uric acid
     D. Ascorbic acid in a dosage of 8 g/day reduces serum uric acid

144. 'Plucked chicken skin' is characteristic of
     A. Pseudoxanthoma elasticum
     B. Ehlers-Danlos syndrome
     C. Osteogenesis imperfecta
     D. Marfan's syndrome

Ans: 138-A 139-B 140-A 141-C 142-B 143-C 144-A

11

Dermatology

1. **Most dangerous type of pemphigus is**
   - A. Pemphigus erythematosus
   - B. Pemphigus foliaceus
   - C. Pemphigus vulgaris
   - D. Pemphigus vegetans

2. **Grattage test is positive in**
   - A. Pemphigus
   - B. Dermatitis herpetiformis
   - C. Psoriasis
   - D. Exfoliative dermatitis

3. **Koebner's phenomenon is found in all *except***
   - A. Pemphigus
   - B. Viral wart
   - C. Lichen planus
   - D. Psoriasis

4. **Tzanck test is negative in**
   - A. HIV
   - B. Herpes zoster
   - C. Varicella
   - D. Herpes simplex

5. **Which is not systemic antifungal agent**
   - A. Flucytosine
   - B. Ketoconazole
   - C. Griseofulvin
   - D. Clotrimazole

6. **Darier's sign is found in**
   - A. Atopic eczema
   - B. Psoriasis
   - C. Pemphigus
   - D. Urticaria pigmentosa

7. **Subepidermal vesicle is seen in**
   - A. Herpes zoster
   - B. Pemphigus
   - C. Herpes simplex
   - D. Bullous pemphigoid

8. **Incidence of vitiligo is increased in all *except***
   - A. Pernicious anaemia
   - B. Acromegaly
   - C. Addison's disease
   - D. Hyperthyroidism

9. **Which is not an antifungal agent**
   - A. Miltefosine
   - B. Flucytosine
   - C. Tolnaftate
   - D. Econazole

Ans: 1-C 2-C 3-A 4-A 5-D 6-D 7-D 8-B 9-A

10. **All of the following drugs cause hyperpigmentation** *except*
    - A. Clofazimine
    - B. INH
    - C. 5-fluorouracil
    - D. Allopurinol

11. **Which histological term is most characteristic for pemphigus**
    - A. Hyperkeratosis
    - B. Acantholysis
    - C. Acanthosis
    - D. Parakeratosis

12. **Pretibial myxoedema is classically found in**
    - A. Subclinical hypothyroidism
    - B. Myxoedema
    - C. Graves' disease
    - D. Hashimoto's thyroiditis

13. **Acne may be produced by all of the following** *except*
    - A. Corticosteroids
    - B. Iodides
    - C. Tetracyclines
    - D. Troxidone

14. **All of the following lesions are found characteristically in front of legs** *except*
    - A. Pretibial myxoedema
    - B. Lupus vulgaris
    - C. Erythema nodosum
    - D. Necrobiosis lipoidica diabeticorum

15. **Photodermatitis is not found in**
    - A. Phenothiazines
    - B. Tetracyclines
    - C. Sulphonamides
    - D. Barbiturates

16. **Cataract may develop in**
    - A. Atopic dermatitis
    - B. Exfoliative dermatitis
    - C. Panniculitis
    - D. Erythema multiforme

17. **Erythema nodosum may be found in therapy by all** *except*
    - A. Penicillin
    - B. Quinolones
    - C. Sulphonamides
    - D. Oral contraceptives

18. **Nicolsky's sign is characteristically positive in**
    - A. Bullous pemphigoid
    - B. Chickenpox
    - C. Pemphigus
    - D. Pityriasis rosea

19. **Stevens-Johnson syndrome is classically seen in all** *except*
    - A. Carbamazepine
    - B. Cotrimoxazole
    - C. Corticosteroids
    - D. Thiacetazones

Ans: 10-D 11-B 12-C 13-C 14-B 15-D 16-A 17-B 18-C 19-C

20. **Comedones are found in**
    A. Seborrhoeic dermatitis   B. Acne vulgaris
    C. Ringworm   D. Vitiligo

21. **Periungual telangiectasia are classically seen in**
    A. SLE
    B. Hereditary haemorrhagic telangiectasia
    C. Acanthosis nigricans
    D. Ataxia telangiectasia

22. **Setvens-Johnson syndrome may be seen in infection caused by**
    A. *Pseudomonas pyocyaneous*
    B. *Streptococcus haemolyticus*
    C. *Staphylococcus aureus*
    D. *Mycoplasma pneumoniae*

23. **A white frontal forelock is found in**
    A. Tuberous sclerosis   B. Addison's disease
    C. Piebaldism   D. Pityriasis alba

24. **Cafe-au-lait spots are characteristically seen in all *except***
    A. Albright's disease   B. Tuberous sclerosis
    C. Neurofibromatosis   D. Friedreich's ataxia

25. **Generalised pruritus may be found in all *except***
    A. Hodgkin's disease   B. Carcinoid syndrome
    C. Haemolytic jaundice   D. Chronic renal failure

26. **'Perifollicufar purpura' is almost pathognomonic of**
    A. Vasculitis   B. Cushing's syndrome
    C. Senile purpura   D. Scurvy

27. **'Target' or 'iris' lesion in skin is characteristic of**
    A. Erythema multiforme   B. Pityriasis rosea
    C. Erythema marginatum   D. Eczema herpeticum

28. **Wornoff rings are seen in**
    A. Acne vulgaris   B. Psoriasis
    C. Ringworm   D. Neurofibromatosis

29. **Palpable purpura may be found in all *except***
    A. Staphylococcaemia   B. Secondary syphilis
    C. Gonococcaemia   D. Meningococcaemia

Ans: 20-B 21-A 22-D 23-C 24-D 25-C 26-D 27-A 28-B 29-B

30. **Hypomelanosis is found in therapy by all** *except*
    - A. Bleomycin
    - B. Hydroquinone
    - C. Corticosteroid
    - D. Retinoic acid

31. **Most pathognomonic lesion in scabies is**
    - A. Vesicles
    - B. Burrow
    - C. Impetigo
    - D. Papules

32. **Pitting nail is found in all** *except*
    - A. Psoriasis
    - B. Alopecia areata
    - C. Eczema
    - D. Urticaria pigmentosa

33. **Acrochordons are**
    - A. Small angiokeratomas
    - B. Same as milia
    - C. Simple skin tags
    - D. Senile lentigo

34. **Norwegian scabies is found in association with all** *except*
    - A. Schizophrenia
    - B. Lepromatous leprosy
    - C. Secondary syphilis
    - D. Down's syndrome

35. **'Perleche' in the angle of the mouth is found in all** *except*
    - A. Ill-fitted dentures
    - B. Candidiasis
    - C. Secondary syphilis
    - C. Leprosy

36. **All of the following lesions are classically 'itchy'** *except*
    - A. Lichen planus
    - B. Dermatitis herpetiformis
    - C. Scabies
    - D. Lupus vulgaris

37. **Pigmentation in Peutz-Jeghers syndrome is characteristically**
    - A. Perioral
    - B. Periumbilical
    - C. In the knuckles of hands
    - D. In the malar prominences

38. **Auspitz's sign is characteristic of**
    - A. Pemphigus
    - B. Discoid lupus erythematosus
    - C. Psoriasis
    - D. Viral wart

39. **Acanthosis nigricans may be associated with all** *except*
    - A. Urticaria pigmentosa
    - B. Diabetes mellitus
    - C. Addison's disease
    - D. Carcinoma of the stomach

Ans: 30-A 31-B 32-D 33-C 34-C 35-D 36-D 37-A 38-C 39-A

40. **All are scabicidal drugs** *except*

   A. Ivermectin
   B. Permethrin
   C. Dithranol
   D. Crotamiton

41. **A big macule is known as**

   A. Papule
   B. Plaque
   C. Patch
   D. Nodule

42. **Calcinosis is found in all of the following** *except*

   A. CREST syndrome
   B. Dermatomyositis
   C. SLE
   D. Scleroderma

43. **Which is not a scaly lesion in skin**

   A. Contact dematitis
   B. Seborrhoeic dermatitis
   C. Exfoliative dermatitis
   D. Ringworm

44. **Lupus-like picture is characteristic of therapy by all** *except*

   A. Chloroquine
   B. Procainamide
   C. INH
   D. Hydralazine

45. **Histoid leprosy is a variety of**

   A. Lepromatous leprosy
   B. Borderline leprosy
   C. Tuberculoid leprosy
   D. Indeterminate leprosy

46. **Chloroquine is indicated in the management of**

   A. Lupus vulgaris
   B. Bullous pemphigoid
   C. Dicsoid lupus erythematosus
   D. Psoriasis

47. **Which is an allergic reaction of primary pulmonary tuberculosis**

   A. Erythema marginatum
   B. Erythema nodosum
   C. Erythema induratum
   D. Erythema multiforme

48. **The drug of choice in dermatitis herpetiformis is**

   A. Ivermectin
   B. Corticosteroids
   C. Dithranol
   D. Dapsone

49. **Erythema nodosum leprosum is classically treated by**

   A. Aspirin
   B. Thalidomide
   C. Chloroquine
   D. Dapsone

Ans: 40-C 41-C 42-C 43-A 44-A 45-A 46-C 47-B 48-D 49-B

50. **Herald patch is characteristically seen in**
    A. Pityriasis alba
    B. Pityriasis versicolor
    C. Pityriasis rosea
    D. Xeroderma pigmentosum

51. **Cicatrical alopecia is seen in all *except***
    A. Lichen planus
    B. Discoid lupus erythematosus
    C. Morphoea
    D. Alopecia areata

52. **Nodular cystic acne is treated with**
    A. Tetracycline
    B. Iso-retinoin
    C. Radiation
    D. Surgery

53. **Flaky paint dermatosis is a feature of**
    A. Pellagra
    B. Marasmus
    C. Scleroderma
    D. Kwashiorkor

54. **Acrodermatitis enteropathica is due to deficiency of**
    A. Manganese
    B. Selenium
    C. Chromium
    D. Zinc

55. **Photochemotherapy is adopted in**
    A. Psoriasis
    B. Exfoliative dermatitis
    C. Lichen planus
    D. Seborrhoeic dermatitis

56. **Erythema nodosum leprosum occurs in**
    A. Borderline tuberculoid leprosy
    B. Tuberculoid leprosy
    C. Neuritic leprosy
    D. Lepromatous leprosy

57. **Hyperpigmentation is not characteristic of**
    A. Addison's disease
    B. Myxoedema
    C. Graves' disease
    D. Cushing's syndrome

58. **All of the following are features of lepromatous leprosy *except***
    A. Collapse of bridge of the nose
    B. Gynaecomastia
    C. Pleurisy
    D. Madarosis

59. **Tinea versicolor is caused by**
    A. *Microsporum*
    B. *Malassezia furfur*
    C. *Epidermophyton*
    D. *Trichophyton*

Ans: 50-C 51-D 52-B 53-D 54-D 55-A 56-D 57-B 58-C 59-B

60. **Erythema nodosum does not occur in**
    A. Primary tuberculosis
    B. Ulcerative colitis
    C. Giant cell arteritis
    D. Sarcoidosis

61. **'Red lunula' in nails is characteristic of**
    A. Ringworm
    B. Discoid lupus erythematosus
    C. Congestive cardiac failure
    D. Chronic renal failure

62. **Commonest site of involvement in atopic dermatitis is**
    A. Flexural areas
    B. Extensor surfaces
    C. Exposed part
    D. Areas of pressure and friction

63. **Discoid lupus erythematosus is not featured by**
    A. Scaling with atrophy
    B. Acanthosis
    C. Telangiectasia
    D. Keratotic plugging

64. **Most potent drug for *Mycobacterium leprae* is**
    A. Clofazimine
    B. Dapsone
    C. Rifampicin
    D. Ofloxacin

65. **Splinter haemorrhage in nails is caused by all *except***
    A. Polycythaemia vera
    B. Subacute bacterial endocarditis
    C. Systemic vasculitis
    D. Trichinosis

66. **Mucous membrane lesions are seen in**
    A. Pemphigoid
    B. Dermatitis herpetiformis
    C. Impetigo
    D. Pemphigus

67. **Palmar erythema is found in all *except***
    A. Pregnancy
    B. Hepatocellular failure
    C. In some normal persons
    D. Hypothyroidism

68. **Characteristic nail change of lichen planus is**
    A. Pitting
    B. Onycholysis
    C. Pterygium
    D. Subungual hyperkeratosis

69. **Erythema marginatum is a feature of**
    A. Sulphonamide therapy
    B. Acute rheumatic fever
    C. Primary tuberculosis
    D. Leprosy

Ans: 60-C 61-C 62-A 63-B 64-C 65-A 66-D 67-D 68-C 69-B

70. **Virchow's cells are seen in**
    A. Leprosy
    B. Toxic epidermal necrolysis
    C. Herpes zoster infection
    D. Henoch-Schonlein purpura

71. **Erythrasma is caused by**
    A. *Staphylococcus aureus*
    B. *Corynebacterium minutissimum*
    C. *Propionibacterium acne*
    D. Vaccinia virus

72. **Leuconychia is a manifestation of**
    A. Iron deficiency anaemia
    B. Bronchogenic carcinoma
    C. Psoriasis
    D. Hypoalbuminaemia

73. **Dermographism is characteristic of**
    A. Ectodermal dysplasia
    B. Xeroderma pigmentosum
    C. Urticaria pigmentosa
    D. Dermatitis herpetiformis

74. **Molluscum contagiosum is caused by**
    A. Poxvirus
    B. Paramyxovirus
    C. Papovavirus
    D. Herpes virus

75. **Rosacea is characterised by all *except***
    A. Usually affects middle-aged females
    B. Corticosteroid therapy may precipitate the condition
    C. May be associated with exposure to cold or strong sunshine
    D. Often exaggerated by consumption of tea

76. **Erythroderma (exfoliative dermatitis) is featured by all *except***
    A. Pemphigus
    B. Eczema
    C. Pityriasis rubra pilaris
    D. Psoriasis

77. **All are features of ringworm *except***
    A. Central clearing
    B. Non-itchy
    C. Active border
    D. Circinate lesion

78. **Which of the following is true regarding lupus vulgaris**
    A. Immune status of the host is at fault
    B. Apple-jelly nodules
    C. Non-scaly in nature
    D. Circular in shape

Ans: 70-A 71-B 72-D 73-C 74-A 75-B 76-A 77-B 78-B

79. **Dermatophytosis does not manifest as**

    A. Tinea versicolor
    B. Tinea cruris
    C. Tinea unguium
    D. Tinea capitis

80. **Kerion is associated with**

    A. Psoriasis
    B. Lichen planus
    C. Discoid lupus erythematosus
    D. Tinea capitis

81. **Dermatitis herpetiformis is**

    A. Intensely pruritic
    B. Common in flexor surfaces
    C. Associated with ulcerative colitis
    D. Treated by corticosteroid

82. **Shagreen patches are classically seen in**

    A. Dermatomyositis
    B. Scleroderma
    C. Tuberous sclerosis
    D. Discoid lupus erythematosus

83. **Fixed drug eruption may be due to all *except***

    A. Ascorbic acid
    B. Phenolphthalein
    C. Barbiturates
    D. Salicylates

84. **Pityriasis alba is featured by all *except***

    A. Worse in summers
    B. Finely scaly
    C. Perhaps infective
    D. Remits spontaneously

85. **Wickham's striae are characteristic of**

    A. Psoriasis
    B. Pemphigus
    C. Dermatitis herpetiformis
    D. Lichen planus

86. **All are true regarding xeroderma pigmentosum *except***

    A. Pre-malignant
    B. Photophobia
    C. Autosomal dominant inheritance
    D. Freckles

87. **Pellagra-like dermatitis may be seen in all *except***

    A. Hartnup disease
    B. Functional carcinoid syndrome
    C. Protein-calorie malnutrition
    D. INH therapy

88. **Shamberg's disease is featured by all *except***

    A. Multiple, brown macules
    B. Most frequently seen in lower legs
    C. Unilateral
    D. Due to capillaritis of unknown aetiology

Ans: 79-A 80-D 81-A 82-C 83-A 84-A 85-D 86-C 87-C 88-C

89. **Discoid lupus erythematosus most commonly affects**
    A. Buccal mucosa
    B. Axilla
    C. Face
    C. Lips

90. **All are true regarding pemphigoid** *except*
    A. May be associated with lymphoma
    B. Large, tense bullae
    C. Little toxaemia
    D. Heals with scarring

91. **Which of the following is not an antifungal agent**
    A. Terbinafine
    B. Itraconazole
    C. Calcipotriol
    D. Griseofulvin

92. **Malignant melanoma usually arises from**
    A. Dermal naevus
    B. Hairy mole
    C. Epidermal naevus
    D. Junctional naevus

93. **Which of the following is false regarding mycosis fungoides**
    A. Non-infiltrative
    B. Cutaneous T-cell lymphoma
    C. Associated with Pautrier's microabscesses in epidermis
    D. Seen in middle-aged or elderly people

94. **Commonest skin infection in children is**
    A. Molluscum contagiosum
    B. Impetigo contagiosa
    C. Viral warts
    D. Scabies

95. **Phrenoderma is due to deficiency of**
    A. Vitamin E
    B. Essential fatty acid
    C. Zinc
    D. Vitamin B_{12}

96. **Rosacea is not associated with**
    A. High sebum secretion
    B. Rhinophyma
    C. Easy flush
    D. Affection of face

97. **Depressed bridge of the nose is found in all** *except*
    A. Ectodermal dysplasia
    B. Cretinism
    C. Tuberculoid leprosy
    D. Wegener's granulomatosis

93. **Gottron's papules are pathognomonic of**
    A. Scleroderma
    B. Discoid lupus erythematosus
    C. Histiocytosis X disease
    D. Dermatomyositis

Ans: 89-C 90-D 91-C 92-D 93-A 94-B 95-B 96-A 97-C 98-D

99. **Heliotrope rash is seen in**
    - A. Progressive systemic sclerosis
    - B. Systemic lupus erythematosus
    - C. Reiter's syndrome
    - D. Deratomyositis

100. **Time taken for a finger nail to form completely**
    - A. 3 months
    - B. 4 months
    - C. 5 months
    - D. 6 months

101. **'Id reaction' is seen in infection with**
    - A. Tuberculosis
    - B. Dermatophytes
    - C. Syphilis
    - D. *Streptococcus*

102. **Sycosis barbae is a disease of**
    - A. Bacterial origin
    - B. Allergic origin
    - C. Viral origin
    - D. Fungal origin

103. **Hidradenitis suppurativa most commonly affects**
    - A. Scalp
    - B. Axilla
    - C. Periumbilical area
    - D. Dorsum of foot

104. **Which of the following is true about pityriasis alba**
    - A. Common in elderly people
    - B. A variant of vitiligo
    - C. Most common over the anterior part of legs
    - D. Heals spontaneously

105. **Acantholysis is characteristic of**
    - A. Dermatitis herpetiformis
    - B. Pemphigus vulgaris
    - C. Psoriasis
    - D. Pemphigoid

106. **The cardinal feature of atopic eczema is**
    - A. Oozing
    - B. Pigmentation
    - C. Itching
    - D. Rash with papules

107. **Which of the following may be tried in chronic urticaria**
    - A. Anti-leukotrienes
    - B. COX-2 inhibitors
    - C. Granulocyte colony stimulating factors
    - D. Anti-prostaglandins

108. **'Pinch purpura' is seen in**
    - A. Epiloia
    - B. Amyloidosis
    - C. von Recklinghausen's disease
    - D. Sideroblastic anaemia

Ans: 99-D 100-C 101-B 102-A 103-B 104-D 105-B 106-C 107-A 108-B

109. Diagnostic test of choice in contact dermatitis is
    A. Intradermal test   B. Tzanck test
    C. Skin biopsy   D. Patch test

110. Which of the following oral ulcers is painless
    A. Behcet's syndrome
    B. Aphthous ulcer
    C. Reiter's syndrome
    D. Stevens-Johnson syndrome

111. Bullous lesion is not characteristic of
    A. Dermatitis herpetiformis   B. Pemphigus
    C. Erythema multiforme   D. Atopic eczema

112. 'Apple-jelly nodule' is characteristic of
    A. Lupus vulgaris
    B. Systemic lupus erythematosus
    C. Lichen planus
    D. Lepromatous leprosy

113. 'Diascopy' is important for diagnosis of all *except*
    A. Purpura   B. Apple-jelly nodule
    C. Pemphigus   D. Telangiectasia

114. Bullous eruptions are characteristic of all *except*
    A. Erythema multiforme
    B. Chronic chloroquine therapy
    C. Barbiturate poisoning
    D. Pemphigoid

115. Mucous membrane involvement does not help in the diagnosis of
    A. Eczema   B. Lichen planus
    C. Erythema multiforme   D. Pemphigus

116. Which of the following has a recognised association with gastrointestinal disorder
    A. Pemphigoid   B. Cafe-au-lait spots
    C. Pyoderma gangrenosum   D. Acne rosacea

117. Exposure to sunlight may aggravate
    A. Psoriasis
    B. Acute intermittent porphyria
    C. Systemic lupus erythematosus
    D. Carotenaemia

Ans: 109-D 110-C 111-D 112-A 113-C 114-B 115-A 116-C 117-C

118. Which of the following is not considered a recognised association
A. Erythema marginatum and acute rheumatic fever
B. Livedo reticularis and antiphospholipid syndrome
C. Acrodermatitis enteropathica and zinc deficiency
D. Pseudoxanthoma elasticum and carcinoma of the colon

119. Ocular signs/symptoms are characteristic of
A. Acne vulgaris B. Rosacea
C. Psoriasis D. Lichen planus

120. Which of the following is not a recognised association
A. Migratory thrombophlebitis and carcinoma of the pancreas
B. Sarcoidosis and lupus pernio
C. Coeliac disease and erythema nodosum
D. AIDS and Kaposi's sarcoma

121. Lichenoid eruptions are not characteristic of
A. Gold salts
B. Quinidine
C. Phenothiazines
D. Chlorpropamide

122. Angioedema may develop as an adverse reaction in therapy with
A. Barbiturates B. Griseofulvin
C. Lithium D. Captopril

123. A positive family history may be obtained in all *except*
A. Dermatitis herpetiformis
B. Angioedema
C. Systemic lupus erythematosus
D. Psoriasis

124. Erythema chronicum migrans is characteristically seen in
A. Lyme's disease
B. Glucagonoma
C. Sarcoidosis
D. Acute rheumatic fever

125. Dennie's line (extra fold of skin beneath lower eyelid) is seen in
A. Myxoedema
B. Atopic dermatitis
C. Amyloidosis
D. Carcinoid syndrome

Ans: 118-D 119-B 120-C 121-B 122-D 123-A 124-A 125-B

126. **Precipitating factors for psoriasis are all *except***
    A. Lithium
    B. Chloroquine
    C. Chlorpromazine
    D. β-blockers

127. **Erythema multiforme may result from infection by**
    A. *Pseudomonas pyocyaneous*
    B. Herpes simplex
    C. *Histoplasma capsulatum*
    D. Vaccinia virus

128. **Lichenoid eruptions may be seen in all *except***
    A. Captopril
    B. Chronic graft versus host disease
    C. Gold salt
    D. Phenytoin

129. **Which of the following results in scarring alopecia**
    A. Telogen effluvium
    B. Alopecia areata
    C. Traumatic alopecia
    D. Lichen planus

130. **Sign of Leser-Trelat does not include**
    A. Endocrinopathy
    B. Acanthosis nigricans
    C. Seborrhoeic keratosis
    D. Acrocordons (skin tags)

131. **Waardenburg's syndrome does not include**
    A. Peibaldism
    B. Sensorineural hearing loss
    C. Heterochromic irises
    D. Hypertelorism

132. **Which of the following is not true regarding Wood's lamp (360 nm uv) examination of skin lesion**
    A. Pseudomonas wounds: Pale blue
    B. Post-inflammatory hyperpigmentation: More black
    C. Tuberous sclerosis: Ash-leaf white spots
    D. Erythrasma: Coral red

133. **Cicatrical alopecia is not due to**
    A. Folliculitis decalvans
    B. Discoid lupus erythematosus
    C. Tinea capitis
    D. Morphea

134. **Incontinentia pigmenti does not have**
    A. X-linked recessive inheritance
    B. Mental retardation
    C. Seizures
    D. Eosinophilia

Ans: 126-C 127-B 128-D 129-D 130-A 131-D 132-B 133-C 134-A

135. **Lofgren's syndrome in sarcoidosis refers to all** *except*

    A. Erythema nodosum
    B. Hilar adenopathy
    C. Acuyte polyarthritis
    D. Malar rash

136. **Violaceous papules may be seen in all** *except*

    A. Lupus pernio
    B. Cutaneous lupus
    C. Lichen planus
    D. Primary amyloidosis

137. **Commonest site of erythema induration is**

    A. Shin   B. Face
    C. Calf   D. Trunk

138. **Nail-patella syndrome may be complicated by**

    A. Ankylosing spondylitis
    B. Cataract
    C. Nephrotic syndrome
    D. Interstitial lung disease

139. **Which one is false regarding bullous pemphigoid**

    A. No association with internal malignancy
    B. Tense bulla
    C. Seen above 60 years of age
    D. Females affected more than males

140. **Atopic dermatitis does not have**

    A. Bullous lesion
    B. Dennie's line (extra fold of skin beneath lower eyelid)
    C. Increased palmar skin markings
    D. Hertogue's sign (thinning of lateral half of eyebrows)

141. **Facial butterfly-rash in SLE is due to**

    A. Increased melanocytic activity
    B. Autoimmune reaction
    C. Apoptosis of keratinized skin layer
    D. Idiopathic

142. **All of the following may cause photodermatoses** *except*

    A. Nalidixic acid   B. Etanercept
    C. Dacarbazine   D. Phenothiazines

Ans: 135-D 136-D 137-C 138-C 139-C 140-A 141-C 142-B

143. Which of the following is not true in Sweet's syndrome
    A. Common in young male subjects
    B. Presents with acute onset of pyrexia and eruption of tender plum-coloured nodule
    C. Episcleritis and oral ulceration are not uncommon
    D. Dramatic response to systemic corticosteroids

144. Typical 'bathing-suit' distribution of skin eruption is characteristic of
    A. Pityriasis rubra pilaris   B. Pityriasis lichenoides chronica
    C. Parapsoriasis   D. Pityriasis rosea

145. Which of the following is not true regarding the facts mentioned below
    A. Average hairs in scalp is more than 100 000
    B. Scalp hair grows 0.3–4 mm/day
    C. 90–95% of hairs are in anagen phase
    D. Up to 10 telogen hairs may be lost per day

146. Which of the following is not a genetic disorder of skin
    A. Dermatitis herpetiformis   B. Ectodermal dysplasia
    C. Tuberous sclerosis   D. Pachydermoperiostosis

12

Rheumatology

1. Which does not produce erythematous butterfly-like lesion in face
   - A. Lupus vulgaris
   - B. Melasma
   - C. SLE
   - D. Scleroderma

2. Which is a recognised pulmonary complication of SLE
   - A. Shrinking lung syndrome
   - B. Caplan's syndrome
   - C. Hidebound chest syndrome
   - D. Pneumoconiosis

3. Which of the following is not associated with active SLE
   - A. High serum level of ANA
   - B. Low serum level of complement
   - C. High serum level of C-reactive protein
   - D. High serum level of anti-ds DNA

4. Which of the following is the specific antibody for SLE
   - A. Anti-Ro/La
   - B. Anti-RNP
   - C. Anti-ss DNA
   - D. Anti-Sm

5. All are characteristic features of DLE *except*
   - A. Photosensitivity
   - B. Telangiectasia
   - C. Raynaud's phenomenon
   - D. Heals with scarring

6. Which of the following is not a recognised complication of SLE
   - A. Diffuse glomerulonephritis
   - B. Membranous nephropathy
   - C. Interstitial nephritis
   - D. Minimal lesion nephropathy

7. Exacerbations of SLE is produced by
   - A. Rifampicin
   - B. Oral contraceptives
   - C. Carbamazepine
   - D. Reserpine

8. Rheumatoid factor in SLE is positive in
   - A. 20% cases
   - B. 35% cases
   - C. 50% cases
   - D. 70% cases

Ans: 1-D 2-A 3-C 4-D 5-C 6-D 7-B 8-A

9. **Which of the following is usually not a skin lesion of SLE**
    A. Panniculitis
    B. Periungual erythema
    C. Erythema nodosum
    D. Bullous lesion

10. **ANF in SLE is positive in approximately**
    A. 60% cases
    B. 70% cases
    C. 80% cases
    D. 95% cases

11. **Lupus nephritis is treated by all *except***
    A. Interferon
    B. Glucocorticoids
    C. Azathioprine
    D. Cyclophosphamide

12. **Progressive systemic sclerosis (PSS) may develop into all *except***
    A. Pulmonary hypertension
    B. Alveolar cell neoplasm
    C. Hypertrophic cardiomyopathy
    D. Heart block

13. **Mixed connective tissue disease (MCTD) is a combination of SLE, scleroderma, rheumatoid arthritis and**
    A. Sjogren's syndrome
    B. Polymyositis
    C. Myasthenia gravis
    D. Osteoarthritis

14. **Raynaud's phenomenon is not a feature of**
    A. Hyperviscosity syndrome
    B. Ergot ingestion
    C. Coarctation of aorta
    D. Dermatomyositis

15. **Mask-like face is seen in all *except***
    A. Depression
    B. Scleroderma
    C. Parkinsonism
    D. Myotonic dystrophy

16. **Pseudoscleroderma is caused by all *except***
    A. Amyloidosis
    B. Cutis laxa
    C. Scleredema
    D. Acromegaly

17. **Raynaud's phenomenon may be treated by**
    A. Methysergide
    B. Propranolol
    C. Naftidrofuryl
    D. Dimethyl sulfoxide

18. **Hands of scleroderma classically may reveal all *except***
    A. Pseudoclubbing
    B. Digital infarcts
    C. Livedo reticularis
    D. Sclerodactyly

Ans: 9-C 10-D 11-A 12-C 13-B 14-C 15-D 16-B 17-C 18-C

19. **All of the following produce mutilated fingers/toes** *except*

    A. Amyloidosis   B. Leprosy
    C. Frostbite   D. Vasculitis

20. **CREST syndrome is aggregation of calcinosis, Raynaud's phenomenon, sclerodactyly, telangiectasia and**

    A. Oedema
    B. Endomyocardial fibrosis
    C. Oesophageal hypomotility
    D. Exophthalmos

21. **HBsAg is present in vasculitis associated with**

    A. Henoch-Schonlein purpura   B. Temporal arteritis
    C. Churg-Strauss syndrome   D. Polyarteritis nodosa

22. **Colchicine may be used in all** *except*

    A. Scleroderma   B. Polymyositis
    C. Myelofibrosis   D. Primary biliary cirrhosis

23. **Polymyalgia rheumatica is not associated with**

    A. Early morning stiffness
    B. Pain in the muscles of neck, shoulder and hip
    C. Elevated muscle enzymes
    D. Very high ESR

24. **In Churg-Strauss syndrome, the principal organ involved is**

    A. Lung   B. Kidney
    C. Central nervous system   D. Liver

25. **Anti-Jo-1 antibody is diagnostic of**

    A. Sjogren's syndrome
    B. Progressive systemic sclerosis
    C. Dermatomyositis with lung disease
    D. Lupus nephritis

26. **Kawasaki disease is associated with**

    A. Coronary artery aneurysm   B. Renal failure
    C. Pleural effusion   D. Hemiplegia

27. **c-ANCA (antinuclear cytoplasmic antibody) is diagnostic of**

    A. Microscopic polyarteritis
    B. Wegener's granulomatosis
    C. Crescentic glomerulonephritis
    D. Polyarteritis nodosa

Ans: 19-A 20-C 21-D 22-B 23-C 24-A 25-C 26-A 27-B

28. **Temporal arteritis is featured by all *except***
    A. Intense headache
    B. May develop permanent blindness
    C. Jaw claudication
    D. Bell's palsy

29. **Anti-RNP antibody is diagnostic of**
    A. MCTD (Sharp's syndrome)
    B. Polymyositis
    C. Drug-induced SLE
    D. Antiphospholipid antibody syndrome

30. **Which organ involvement is not included within the classic triad of Wegener's granulomatosis**
    A. Lower respiratory tract   B. Cardiovascular system
    C. Kidney   D. Upper respiratory tract

31. **Subcutaneous nodules are seen in all *except***
    A. Cysticercosis   B. Leprosy
    C. Dermatomyositis   D. Rheumatic fever

32. **Sero-negative arthropathy is not associated with**
    A. Iritis   B. Sacroiliitis
    C. Mononeuritis multiplex   D. Enthesopathy

33. **Which of the following is not associated with carpal tunnel syndrome**
    A. Acromegaly   B. Primary amyloidosis
    C. Pregnancy   D. Thyrotoxicosis

34. **Hyperostosis may be a complication of systemic therapy with**
    A. Retinoids   B. Sodium fluoride
    C. Calcipotriol   D. Alendronate

35. **Rose-Waaler test (RF) is positive in rheumatoid arthritis in**
    A. 30% cases   B. 45% cases
    C. 70% cases   D. 90% cases

36. **Fibromyalgia is characterised by all *except***
    A. Female preponderance
    B. High CPK
    C. Focal point tenderness
    D. Improvement by tricyclic antidepressant

Ans: 28-D 29-A 30-B 31-C 32-C 33-D 34-A 35-C 36-B

37. **Viscosity of synovial fluid in osteoarthritis is**
    - A. Very low
    - B. High
    - C. Low
    - D. Remains as normal

38. **Calcinosis is featured by all *except***
    - A. Rheumatoid arthritis
    - B. Childhood dermatomyositis
    - C. CREST syndrome
    - D. Scleroderma

39. **Forrestier's disease is associated with**
    - A. Malar rash
    - B. Pulmonary nodules
    - C. Hyperostosis
    - D. Vasculitis

40. **Rheumatoid nodules are characterised by all *except***
    - A. Big
    - B. Tender
    - C. Fixed to skin
    - D. Ulcerate

41. **Classically which of the following does not produce polyarthralgia**
    - A. Depression
    - B. Haemophilia
    - C. Myxoedema
    - D. Fibromyalgia

42. **Still's disease does not give rise to**
    - A. Positive Rose-Waaler test
    - B. Splenomegaly
    - C. Lymphadenopathy
    - D. Maculopapular rash

43. **Bouchard's nodes in osteoarthritis are seen in**
    - A. Carpometacarpal joint
    - B. Metacarpophalangeal joint
    - C. Proximal interphalangeal joint
    - D. Distal interphalangeal joint

44. **Pseudogout (chondrocalcinosis) is associated with deposition of crystals of**
    - A. Calcium oxalate
    - B. Monosodium urate
    - C. Calcium phosphate
    - D. Calcium pyrophosphate dihydrate

45. **All of the following indicate poor prognosis in rheumatoid arthritis *except***
    - A. High titre of rheumatoid factor
    - B. Extra-articular manifestations
    - C. Acute onset of disease
    - D. Early developement of nodules

Ans: 37-B 38-A 39-C 40-B 41-B 42-A 43-C 44-D 45-C

46. Ocular manifestations of rheumatoid arthritis usually do not include
    A. Anterior uveitis
    B. Episcleritis
    C. Keratoconjunctivitis sicca
    D. Scleromalacia

47. Drug of choice for relieving pain in osteoarthritis is
    A. Corticosteroids
    B. Ibuprofen
    C. Paracetamol
    D. Diclofenac

48. Which of the following is not a disease-modifying antirheumatic drug (DMARD)
    A. Hydroxychloroquine sulphate
    B. Leflunomide
    C. Sulphasalazine
    D. Naproxen

49. Pseudogout may result from all except
    A. Gout
    B. Haemochromatosis
    C. Ochronosis
    D. Hyperphosphatasia

50. Felly's syndrome is not associated with
    A. Age of onset 20–25 yrs
    B. Vasculitis
    C. Lymphadenopathy
    D. Thrombocytopenia

51. Polarised light microscopy of synovial fluid in gout shows
    A. Negatively birefringent monosodium urate crystals
    B. Positively birefringent calcium urate crystals
    C. Positively birefringent monosodium urate crystals
    D. Negatively birefringent calcium urate crystals

52. All are extra-articular manifestations of rheumatoid arthritis except
    A. Fibrosing alveolitis
    B. Pericarditis
    C. Mononeuritis multiplex
    D. Ulcerative colitis

53. Reiter's syndrome is not featured by
    A. Circinate balanitis
    B. Subungual hyperkeratosis
    C. Pyoderma gangrenosum
    D. Keratoderma blenorrhagica

54. Angioneurotic oedema may be treated by
    A. Diuretics
    B. Danazol
    C. Mineralocorticoids
    D. Tropical corticosteroid

Ans: 46-A 47-C 48-D 49-D 50-A 51-A 52-D 53-C 54-B

55. **Autoantibody not found in Sjögren's syndrome is**
    A. Anti-La
    B. Salivary duct
    C. Gastric parietal cell
    D. Alveolar cells

56. **Which bacterium is not associated with reactive arthritis**
    A. *Chlamydia*
    B. *Shigella*
    C. *Staphylococcus*
    D. *Campylobacter*

57. **Drug-induced SLE is not commonly associated with**
    A. Polyarthritis
    B. Pulmonary infiltrates
    C. Renal involvement
    D. Polyserositis

58. **Positive 'Dagger sign' in X-ray of spine is a feature of**
    A. Psoriatic arthropathy
    B. Ankylosing spondylitis
    C. Reactive arthritis
    D. Rheumatoid arthritis

59. **'Pathergy' is characteristic of**
    A. Reiter's syndrome
    B. Lyme arthritis
    C. Behçet's syndrome
    D. Leucocytoclastic vasculitis

60. **Asceptic necrosis of bone is not a feature of**
    A. Rheumatoid arthritis
    B. Decompression sickness
    C. Corticosteroid therapy
    D. Sickle-cell disease

61. **Eosinophilic fascitis does not give rise to**
    A. Dysphagia
    B. Eosinophilia
    C. Carpal tunnel syndrome
    D. Hyperglobulinaemia

62. **Which of the following is not an extra-articular manifestation of ankylosing spondylitis**
    A. Acute pulmonary fibrosis
    B. Aortic incompetence
    C. Amyloidosis
    D. Raynaud's phenomenon

63. **Hereditary angioneurotic oedema is due to**
    A. C_1 esterase inhibitor deficiency
    B. Hypocomplementaemia C_2
    C. Deficiency of leukotrienes
    D. Excess of prostaglandin D_2

64. **The most effective prophylaxis adopted in gout by**
    A. Allopurinol
    B. Benzbromarone
    C. Pronbenecid
    D. Colchicine

Ans: 55-D 56-C 57-C 58-B 59-C 60-A 61-A 62-D 63-A 64-A

65. **Lyme arthritis is**
    A. Tick-borne spirochaetal infection
    B. Autoimmune disease
    C. Viral infection
    D. Bacterial infection

66. **Osteosclerosis of the spine may be seen in all** *except*
    A. Osteopetrosis   B. Fluorosis
    C. Hodgkin's disease   D. Osteomalacia

67. **Terminal interphalangeal joint is classically involved in**
    A. Rheumatoid arthritis   B. Reactive arthritis
    C. Behçet's syndrome   D. Psoriatic arthropathy

68. **Clutton's joint is characteristic of**
    A. Congenital syphilis   B. Diabetes mellitus
    C. Tabes dorsalis   D. Chondrocalcinosis

69. **Behçet's syndrome is not associated with**
    A. Meningoencephalitis   B. Genital ulceration
    C. Thrombophlebitis   D. Urethritis

70. **Heberden's node is seen in**
    A. Osteoarthritis   B. Progressive systemic sclerosis
    C. Dermatomyositis   D. Gout

71. **Hypertrophic osteoarthropathy is least common in**
    A. Mesothelioma of pleura B. Bronchogenic carcinoma
    C. Metastatic tumour of lung D. Pachydermoperiostitis

72. **Scleroderma-like lesion may be produced by all** *except*
    A. Vinyl chloride   B. Bleomycin
    C. Hydralazine   D. Pentazocine

73. **All are true regarding causes of Dupuytren's contracture** *except*
    A. Alcoholic cirrhosis
    B. Working with vibrating tools
    C. Progressive systemic sclerosis
    D. Phenytoin therapy in epileptics

74. **Syndesmophytes are seen in all** *except*
    A. Reiter's syndrome   B. Osteopetrosis
    C. Ankylosing spondylitis D. Psoriatic arthritis

Ans: 65-A 66-D 67-D 68-A 69-D 70-A 71-C 72-C 73-C 74-B

75. **Multiple myeloma is associated with all of the following** *except*
    A. Bone pain
    B. Hypercalcaemia
    C. High alkaline phosphatase
    D. Bone marrow failure

76. **HLA-B27 tissue typing is not associated with**
    A. Psoriatic arthropathy
    B. Ankylosing spondylitis
    C. Reiter's syndrome
    D. Behçet's syndrome

77. **Paget's disease is not manifested by**
    A. Coldness of the extremities
    B. Angioid streaks in retina
    C. Spontaneous fracture
    D. High-output cardiac failure

78. **Polyarthritis is the affection of more than**
    A. 1 joint
    B. 2 joints
    C. 3 joints
    D. 4 joints

79. **Which of the following is not a side effect of penicillamine**
    A. Nephrotic syndrome
    B. Myasthenia gravis
    C. Pemphigus
    D. Wilson's disease

80. **Myopathy may develop from all** *except*
    A. Statins
    B. Corticosteroid
    C. Amphotericin B
    D. Glutethimide

81. **Commonest organism involved in osteomyelitis is**
    A. *Salmonella*
    B. Group A β-haemolytic streptococci
    C. *Staphylococcus aureus*
    D. *Mycobacterium tuberculosis*

82. **Which organ involvement does not occur in progressive systemic sclerosis**
    A. Central nervous system
    B. Renal
    C. Cardiac
    D. Pulmonary

83. **Highest incidence of rheumatoid factor (RF) is found in**
    A. SLE
    B. Sjögren's syndrome
    C. Rheumatoid arthritis
    D. Progressive systemic sclerosis

84. **Antitopoisomerase-1 virtually diagnoses**
    A. Wegener's granulomatosis
    B. Sjögren's syndrome
    C. Progressive systemic sclerosis
    D. Juvenile rheumatoid arthritis

Ans: 75-C 76-D 77-A 78-D 79-D 80-D 81-C 82-A 83-B 84-C

85. **TNF-antagonist used in treatment of rheumatoid arthritis is**
   - A. Leflunomide
   - B. Azathioprine
   - C. Etanercept
   - D. Salphasalazine

86. **Oesophagus is most commonly involved by**
   - A. Progressive systemic sclerosis
   - B. Polymyositis
   - C. Polyarteritis nodosa
   - D. Behçet's syndrome

87. **Sjögren's syndrome may be associated with all *except***
   - A. Primary biliary cirrhosis
   - B. SLE
   - C. Myasthenia gravis
   - D. Bronchial asthma

88. **Dystrophic calcinosis is classically seen in**
   - A. Extravasation of calcium salt during injection
   - B. Scleroderma
   - C. Hyperparathyroidism
   - D. Vitamin D toxicity

89. **Hypertrophic osteoarthropathy is most commonly due to**
   - A. Mesothelioma of pleura
   - B. COPD
   - C. Bronchogenic carcinoma
   - D. Fibrosing alveolitis

90. **Example of autoimmune arthritis is**
   - A. Rheumatoid arthritis
   - B. Haemophilic arthritis
   - C. Psoriatic arthritis
   - D. Osteoarthritis

91. **Regarding drug-induced SLE, which is false**
   - A. Nephritis is rare
   - B. Hydralazine and procainamide are most common offenders
   - C. Anti-histone antibodies are present
   - D. Central nervous system involvement is common

92. **Which of the following is commonly involved in Paget's disease**
   - A. Pelvis
   - B. Skull
   - C. Phalanges
   - D. Long bones of extremities

93. **Inhibition of 5-lipoxygenase is beneficial in the treatment of**
   - A. Rheumatoid arthritis
   - B. Hepatorenal syndrome
   - C. Bronchial asthma
   - D. Vasculitis

Ans: 85-C 86-A 87-D 88-B 89-C 90-A 91-D 92-B 93-C

94. Rheumatoid arthritis is strongly associated with histocompatibility antigen
    - A. DR3
    - B. B27
    - C. DR4
    - D. B8

95. A 20-year woman has repeated attacks of myalgia, non-deforming arthralgia, pericarditis and pleural effusion for two years. The laboratory screening test should be
    - A. Rose-Waaler test
    - B. Antinuclear antibodies
    - C. CD4 lymphocyte count
    - D. ASO titre

96. If a patient of scleroderma with Raynaud's phenomenon immerses hand in cold water, the hand will
    - A. Turn red
    - B. Become white
    - C. Turn blue
    - D. Remain unchanged

97. Which is true regarding synovial fluid analysis in osteoarthritis
    - A. High viscosity
    - B. Cloudy in colour
    - C. $4000–8000$ cells/mm^3
    - D. Low complement CH_{50}

98. Which of the following is recognised extra-articular manifestation of ankylosing spondylitis
    - A. Mitral stenosis
    - B. Acute pulmonary fibrosis
    - C. Pericarditis
    - D. Mononeuritis multiplex

99. Eosinophilic fascitis is associated with all *except*
    - A. Eosinophilia
    - B. Raynaud's phenomenon
    - C. Excessive consumption of L-tryptophan
    - D. Usually a self-limiting disease

100. Nodal osteoarthritis is common in
    - A. Hypertension
    - B. Middle-aged females
    - C. Diabetes mellitus
    - D. Gout

101. In rheumatoid arthritis, rheumatoid factor is formed against
    - A. IgG
    - B. IgA
    - C. IgM
    - D. IgD

102. Extra-articular manifestations in rheumatoid arthritis are commonly associated with
    - A. Low C_3
    - B. Females
    - C. High-titre rheumatoid factor
    - D. Delayed age of onset

Ans: 94-C 95-B 96-B 97-A 98-B 99-B 100-B 101-A 102-C

103. **Penicillamine and colchicine both are used in treatment of**
    A. Rheumatoid arthritis
    B. Systemic lupus erythematosus
    C. Progressive systemic sclerosis
    D. Wilson's disease

104. **Hydroxychloroquine toxicity does not produce**
    A. Maculopathy   B. Corneal deposits
    C. Optic atrophy   D. Cataract

105. **False-positive serological test (VDRL) persisting for 6 months is seen in all** *except*
    A. Yaws   B. Leprosy
    C. Antiphospholipid syndrome   D. Glandular fever

106. **Recurrent anterior uveitis is most characteristic of**
    A. Behçet's syndrome
    B. Rheumatoid arthritis
    C. Systemic lupus erythematosus
    D. Sjögren's syndrome

107. **Cytoid (colloid) bodies in the retina is recognised finding in**
    A. Cranial arteritis
    B. Retinal vein thrombosis
    C. Systemic lupus erythematosus
    D. Reiter's syndrome

108. **Still's disease is classically associated with all** *except*
    A. Sacroiliitis
    B. Maculopapular rash
    C. Negative Rose-Waaler test
    D. Involvement of metacarpophalangeal joints

109. **Commonest metabolic bone disease is**
    A. Osteoarthritis   B. Rickets
    C. Osteoporosis   D. Osteomalacia

110. **Avascular necrosis of bone is a recognised association in all** *except*
    A. Sickle-cell disease   B. Parachute diving
    C. Cushing's syndrome   D. Post-renal transplant

111. **Osteomalacia may be produced by therapy with all** *except*
    A. Phenytoin   B. Glucocorticoids
    C. Isoniazid   D. Ketoconazole

Ans: 103-C 104-D 105-D 106-A 107-C 108-A 109-C 110-B 111-B

112. **Polyarteritis nodosa is not manifested by**
    A. Mononeuritis multiplex   B. Asthma
    C. HbsAg positivity   D. Erythema nodosum

113. **Hyperostosis is seen in all** *except*
    A. Hyperthyroidism   B. Paget's disease
    C. Acromegaly   D. Primary hyperparathyroidisrn

114. **Which is false in rheumatoid arthritis so far as ARA criteria is concerned**
    A. Rheumatoid nodules   B. Asymmetrical arthritis
    C. Morning stiffness >1 hour   D. Arthritis of hand joints

115. **Rheumatoid arthritis patients confront an increased risk of developing all** *except*
    A. Hodgkin's disease   B. Leukaemia
    C. Gastrointestinal malignancy D. Non-Hodgkin's lymphoma

116. **Which is not true in pleural disease of rheumatoid arthritis**
    A. Exudative effusion   B. Glucose 10–50 mg/dl
    C. High CH_{50} D. Protein > 4 g/dl

117. **'Arthritis mutilans' is characteristic of**
    A. Psoriasis   B. Reiter's syndrome
    C. Behçet's syndrome   D. Sjögren's syndrome

118. **CREST syndrome is diagnosed by the presence of**
    A. Anti-RNP antibody   B. Anti-centromere antibody
    C. Anti-Jo-1 antibody   D. Anti-histone antibody

119. **Which type of collagen is abundant in bones**
    A. Type IV   B. Type II
    C. Type III   D. Type I

120. **Onion-skin spleen is classically seen in**
    A. Scleroderma
    B. Systemic lupus erythematosus
    C. Mixed connective tissue disease
    D. Sjögren's syndrome

121. **Drug-induced livedo reticularis is seen with**
    A. Amiodarone   B. Finasteride
    C. Amantadine   D. Bromocryptine

Ans: 112-D 113-A 114-B 115-C 116-C 117-A 118-B 119-D 120-B 121-C

122. **Brucella arthritis commonly affects**
    A. Knee joint
    B. Joints of hands
    C. Spine
    D. Metatarsophalangeal joint

123. **Sneddon's syndrome in antiphospholipid syndrome has skin manifestation as**
    A. Livedo reticularis
    B. Nail-fold thrombi
    C. Erythema nodosum
    D. Palpable purpura

124. **False-positive lupus band test is seen in all *except***
    A. Rosacea
    B. Porphyria cutanea tarda
    C. Mixed connective tissue disease
    D. Rheumatoid arthritis

125. **Metacarpophalangeal joints are usually not affected in**
    A. Osteoarthritis
    B. Reactive arthritis
    C. Ankylosing spondylitis
    D. Rheumatoid arthritis

126. **Which of the following usually presents as monoarthropathy**
    A. SLE
    B. Rheumatoid arthritis
    C. Gout
    D. Sjögren's syndrome

127. **Anti-cytokine therapy is usually not associated with**
    A. Demyelination
    B. Anaphylaxis
    C. Reactivation of latent tuberculosis
    D. Reversible lupus-syndrome

128. **Jaccoud's arthropathy is not characteristic of**
    A. Sarcoidosis
    B. Reiter's syndrome
    C. Rheumatic fever
    D. Systemic lupus erythematosus

129. **ANF is not found in SLE, when there is**
    A. Overlap syndrome
    B. Presence of lupus anticoagulant
    C. Chronic renal failure
    D. Presence of anti-cardiolipin antibody

130. **All of the following rheumatological disorders are commonly encountered in diabetes mellitus *except***
    A. Dupuytren's contracture
    B. Cheiroarthropathy
    C. Osteoarthritis of knee
    D. Sacroiliitis

Ans: 122-C 123-A 124-B 125-A 126-C 127-B 128-B 129-C 130-D

131. **Which is not used to treat acute gouty arthritis**
    A. Etoricoxib
    B. Allopurinol
    C. Prednisolone
    D. Colchicine

132. **Finkelstein's test is positive in**
    A. De Quervains' tenosynovitis
    B. Cervical rib
    C. Dupuytren's contracture
    D. Ankylosing spondylitis

133. **Which of the following is not regarded as a 'small vessel' vasculitides**
    A. Microscopic polyangiitis
    B. Henoch-Schönlein purpura
    C. Polyarteritis nodosa
    D. Essential mixed cryoglobulinaemia

134. **Which of the following is false regarding anti-cyclic citrullinated peptide (CCP) antibody**
    A. Commonly found in rheumatoid arthritis
    B. Present in approximately 1.5% of normal population
    C. Common in non-smokers
    D. Psoriatic arthropathy patients may have anti-CCP positivity

135. **Gout may be treated by all *except***
    A. Interleukin-1 inhibitor, anakinra
    B. Benzbromarone
    C. Pegloticase
    D. Olmesartan

Ans: 131-B 132-A 133-C 134-C 135-D

13

Endocrinology

1. **Features of hypoglycaemia do not include**
   A. Drenching sweat   B. Tachycardia
   C. Tachypnoea   D. Brisk jerk

2. **Earliest changes observed by ophthalmoscope in background retinopathy of diabetes is**
   A. Venous dilatation
   B. Microaneurysms
   C. Increased capillary permeability
   D. Arteriovenous shunts

3. **Which of the following is not a part of metabolic 'syndrome X'**
   A. Hyperlipidaemia   B. Obesity
   C. Ischaemic heart disease   D. Hypertension

4. **Thiazolidinedione group of antidiabetic is**
   A. Voglibose   B. Nateglinide
   C. Rosiglitazone   D. Glimepiride

5. **Effect of diabetes on foetus includes all *except***
   A. Microsomia   B. Hyperbilirubinaemia
   C. Stillbirth   D. Open neural tube defect

6. **All are features of diabetic ketoacidosis *except***
   A. Hyperthermia   B. Drowsiness
   C. Dehydration   D. Air hunger

7. **Commonest cause of coma in a diabetic is**
   A. Diabetic ketoacidosis
   B. Lactic acidosis
   C. Hyperosmolar non-ketotic coma
   D. Hypoglycaemia

Ans: 1-C 2-B 3-C 4-C 5-A 6-A 7-D

8. **Which of the following is not a feature of diabetes mellitus**

   A. Rubeosis iridis   B. Pseudo Argyll Robertson pupil
   C. Hippus   D. Isolated IIIrd cranial nerve palsy

9. **A patient of impaired fasting glucose ranges blood glucose value in between**

   A. 96–106 mg/dl   B. 106–116 mg/dl
   C. 100–125 mg/dl   D. 116–130 mg/dl

10. **Glycated fructosamine gives an indication of glycaemia control for last**

   A. 3 days   B. 7 days
   C. 10 days   D. 14 days

11. **Neurological features of myxoedema include all of the following *except***

   A. Delayed relaxation of ankle jerk
   B. Cerebellar ataxia
   C. Hypertonia
   D. Bradylalia

12. **Hypoglycaemia may result from all *except***

   A. Glycogen storage disease   B. Chronic pancreatitis
   C. Galactosaemia   D. Post-gastrectomy

13. **Which of the following is not a neuromuscular feature of thyrotoxicosis**

   A. Myasthenic syndrome
   B. Brisk knee jerk
   C. Hypokalaemic periodic paralysis
   D. Hyperkinesia

14. **Myxoedema coma is characterised by**

   A. Hypertension   B. Tachycardia
   C. Euthermia   D. Hypoventilation

15. **Commonest cause of unilateral exophthalmos is**

   A. Cavernous sinus thrombosis B. Retrobulbar tumour
   C. Chloroma   D. Thyrotoxicosis

16. **Thyroid eye disease is treated by all *except***

   A. 1% methyl cellulose   B. Prednisolone
   C. 5% guanidine   D. Levothyroxine

17. **'Microalbuminuria' is urinary albumin excretion ratio**

   A. 10–100 µg/min   B. 20–200 µg/min
   C. 30–300 µg/min   D. 40–400 µg/min

Ans: 8-C 9-C 10-D 11-C 12-B 13-B 14-D 15-D 16-D 17-B

18. **Hypothyroidism in neonatal period is manifested by all** *except*
    A. Prolonged physiological jaundice
    B. Hoarse cry
    C. Diarrhoea
    D. Somnolence

19. **Sleeping pulse rate is not increased in**
    A. Anxiety neurosis   B. Rheumatic carditis
    C. Pulmonary tuberculosis   D. Atropinised patient

20. **Which of the following is not a feature of autonomic neuropathy in diabetes**
    A. Retrograde ejaculation
    B. Gustatory sweating
    C. Mononeuritis multiplex
    D. Hypoglycaemic unresponsiveness

21. **Beta-blockers can be used in all** *except*
    A. Glaucoma   B. Bronchial asthma
    C. Anxiety states   D. Angina pectoris

22. **Cardiovascular findings of thyrotoxicosis do not include**
    A. Loud S_1 B. Means-Lerman scartch
    C. Water-hammer pulse   D. Ejection click

23. **Myxoedema is characterised by all** *except*
    A. Butterfly rash in face   B. Sinus bradycardia
    C. Solid oedema   D. Madarosis

24. **Secondary hypothyroidism is not featured by**
    A. Normal cholesterol   B. Menorrhagia
    C. Low TSH   D. Fine hairs

25. **Thyroid acropachy is found in**
    A. Subclinical hypothyroidism   B. Graves' disease
    C. Myxoedema   D. Medullary carcinoma of thyroid

26. **Upper segment > lower segment of body is found in all (in dwarfism)** *except*
    A. Pituitary dwarf   B. Cretinism
    C. Achondroplasia   D. Juvenile myxoedema

27. **Acromegaly is associated with all of the following** *except*
    A. Acanthosis nigricans   B. Fibromata mollusca
    C. Micrognathia   D. Cardiomegaly

Ans: 18-C 19-A 20-C 21-B 22-D 23-A 24-B 25-B 26-A 27-C

28. **Klinefelter's syndrome is characterised by**
    A. Small, soft testes
    B. Chromosomal pattern 46, XO
    C. Upper segment > lower segment of body
    D. Gynaecomastia

29. **Which of the following is not an intermediate-acting glucocorticoid**
    A. Cortisone
    B. Triamcinolone
    C. Prednisolone
    D. Prednisone

30. **Hirsutism may develop from all** *except*
    A. Psoralens
    B. Diazoxide
    C. Carbamazepine
    D. Minoxidil

31. **Tall stature is not characteristic of**
    A. Klinefelter's syndrome
    B. Homocystinuria
    C. Marfan's syndrome
    D. Turner's syndrome

32. **Which cranial nerve is not involved in acromegaly**
    A. VIII
    B. III, IV, VI
    C. V
    D. II

33. **Cushing's syndrome does not give rise to**
    A. Hirsutism
    B. Peripheral neuropathy
    C. Purple striae
    D. Acne

34. **Medical adrenalectomy is done by all** *except*
    A. Aminoglutethimide
    B. Mitotane
    C. Mexiletine
    D. Metyrapone

35. **'Pseudo-Cushing's syndrome' may be found in all** *except*
    A. Myxoedema
    B. Chronic alcoholism
    C. Obesity
    D. Depression

36. **Sheehan's syndrome presents with**
    A. Cardiac failure
    B. Persistent lactation
    C. Fever
    D. Striking cachexia

37. **Hypocalcaemia is produced by all** *except*
    A. Hysterical hypoventilation
    B. Acute pancreatitis
    C. Chronic renal failure
    D. Osteomalacia

Ans: 28-D 29-A 30-C 31-D 32-C 33-B 34-C 35-A 36-D 37-A

38 'Menopause' may be manifested by all *except*
  - A. Hirsutism
  - B. Emotional lability
  - C. Osteoporosis
  - D. Phobic neuroses

39. Gynaecomastia may be produced after treatment with all *except*
  - A. Spironolactone
  - B. Digitalis
  - C. Cimetidine
  - D. Rifampicin

40 Primary hyperaldosteronism is not featured by
  - A. Diastolic hypertension
  - B. Paraesthesia
  - C. Alkalosis
  - D. Oedema

41. Thyrotoxicosis may be featured by all *except*
  - A. Myopathy
  - B. Pretibial myxoedema
  - C. Hypernatraemia
  - D. Atrial fibrillation

42. Which of the following is not associated with hypothyroidism
  - A. Loss of libido
  - B. Weight loss
  - C. Cardiac failure
  - D. Organic pyschosis

43. Tetany is characterised by all of the following signs *except*
  - A. Trousseau's sign
  - B. Tinel's sign
  - C. Erb's sign
  - D. Peroneal sign

44. All of the following are featured by dermal hyperpigmentation *except*
  - A. Conn's syndrome
  - B. Bronchogenic carcinoma
  - C. Addison's disease
  - D. Haemochromatosis

45. Hyperparathyroidism is not featured by
  - A. Acute pancreatitis
  - B. Nephrocalcinosis
  - C. Palpable neck swelling
  - D. Pseudogout

46. Phaeochromocytoma is not associated with
  - A. Weight gain
  - B. Fear of death (angor animi)
  - C. Paroxysmal hypertension
  - D. Constipation

47. Which of the following is false regarding medullary carcinoma of thyroid
  - A. Cervical lymphadenopathy
  - B. High serum calcitonin
  - C. Carcinoid syndrome may be associated with
  - D. Psychosis

Ans: 38-D 39-D 40-D 41-C 42-B 43-B 44-A 45-C 46-A 47-D

48. **Malignant hypercalcaemia is treated by all *except***
    A. Pamidronate
    B. Calcitonin
    C. Calcitriol
    D. Glucocorticoids

49. **Most common type of carcinoma of the thyroid gland is**
    A. Follicular
    B. Anaplastic
    C. Papillary
    D. Mixed (A+C)

50. **Features of Addison's disease do not include**
    A. Diarrhoea
    B. Dizziness
    C. Dermatitis
    D. Dehydration

51. **Pseudohypoparathyroidism is not associated with**
    A. Cataract
    B. Raised level of plasma PTH
    C. Mental retardation
    D. Reduced level of plasma phosphate

52. **Commonest cause of phaeochromocytoma is**
    A. Tumour of adrenal medulla
    B. Necrosis of adrenal gland
    C. Small cell carcinoma of bronchus
    D. Adrenal cortical hyperplasia

53. **Commonest cause of Addison's disease is**
    A. Granuloma
    B. Idiopathic atrophy
    C. Inflammatory necrosis
    D. Malignancy

54. **All of the following are noted in Cushing's syndrome *except***
    A. Psychosis
    B. Systemic hypertension
    C. Sexual precocity
    D. Osteoporosis

55. **Secondary hyperaldosteronism is associated with all *except***
    A. Congestive cardiac failure
    B. Nephrotic syndrome
    C. SIADH
    D. Cirrhosis of liver

56. **Empty sella syndrome may be due to all *except***
    A. Sheehan's syndrome
    B. Spontaneous development
    C. Pituitary tumour
    D. Post-irradiation necrosis of pituitary gland

Ans: 48-C 49-D 50-C 51-D 52-A 53-B 54-C 55-C 56-C

57. **Increased muscle mass with slowness of activity (Hoffman syndrome) is seen in**
    A. Acromegaly
    B. Myxoedema
    C. Pseudohypoparathyroidism
    D. Myotonia dystrophica

58. **All of the following develop into dwarfism** *except*
    A. Congenital adrenal hyperplasia
    B. Hypopituitarism
    C. Homocystinuria
    D. Pseudohypoparathyroidism

59. **Plummer's nails are a feature of**
    A. Atopic eczema
    B. Hypoparathyroidism
    C. Thyrotoxicosis
    D. Multiple endocrine neoplasia-type I

60. **Froehlich's syndrome is characterised by all** *except*
    A. Infantilism
    B. Truncal obesity
    C. Diabetes mellitus
    D. Mental retardation

61. **The triad of hyponatraemia, haemodilution and urine hypertonic to plasma suggest diagnosis of**
    A. Nephrotic syndrome
    B. SIADH
    C. Nephrogenic diabetes insipidus
    D. Addison's disease

62. **'Heel-pad thickness' for a male acromegaly should be**
    A. > 14 mm
    B. > 18 mm
    C. > 19 mm
    D. > 21 mm

63. **Nephrogenic diabetes insipidus may develop due to all** *except*
    A. Cystinosis
    B. Lithium-induced
    C. Chronic hepatitis
    D. Heavy metal poisoning

64. **All of the following drugs may produce galactorrhoea** *except*
    A. Salicylates
    B. Reserpine
    C. Cimetidine
    D. Methyldopa

65. **All of the following produce hypergonadotropic hypogonadism** *except*
    A. Sertoli cell only tumour
    B. Klinefelter's syndrome
    C. Kallman's syndrome
    D. Reifenstein's syndrome

Ans: 57-B 58-C 59-C 60-C 61-B 62-D 63-C 64-A 65-C

66. **Which is not a part of multiple endocrine neoplasia-type I (Wermer's syndrome)**
    A. Phaeochromocytoma
    B. Tumour of pituitary
    C. Tumour of pancreas
    D. Hyperparathyroidism

67. **Calcification of basal ganglia is seen in**
    A. Primary hyperparathyroidism
    B. Hypoparathyroidism
    C. Secondary hyperparathyroidism
    D. Milk-alkali syndrome

68. **Phaeochromocytoma may be associated with following anomalies** *except*
    A. Neurofibromatosis
    B. Medullary carcinoma of thyroid
    C. Hyperparathyroidism
    D. Addison's disease

69. **Tertiary hyperparathyroidism is commonly found in**
    A. Rickets
    B. Pseudohypoparathyroidism
    C. Chronic renal failure
    D. Malabsorption syndrome

70. **Commonest enzymatic defect for development of congenital adrenal hyperplasia is**
    A. C-21 hydroxylase deficiency
    B. 3β dehydrogenase deficiency
    C. C-11 hydroxylase deficiency
    D. C-17 hydroxylase deficiency

71. **'Brown tumour' of bone is found in**
    A. Primary hyperparathyroidism
    B. Pseudohypoparathyroidism
    C. Secondary hyperparathyroidism
    D. Hypoparathyroidism

72. **Primary aldosteronism is not featured by**
    A. Low plasma renin
    B. Hypokalaemia
    C. Oedema
    D. Systemic hypertension

73. **Which is not a feature of mucosal neuroma syndrome (multiple endocrine neoplasia-type III)**
    A. Cafe-au-lait spots
    B. Blubbery lips
    C. Kyphoscoliosis
    D. Thickened ulnar nerve

74. **Necrolytic migratory erythema is characteristic of**
    A. Insulinoma
    B. Zollinger-Ellison syndrome
    C. Pancreatic cholera
    D. Glucagonoma

Ans: 66-A 67-B 68-D 69-C 70-A 71-A 72-C 73-D 74-D

75. **Prader-Willi syndrome is featured by all** *except*
    A. Mental retardation
    B. Obesity
    C. Hypertonia
    D. Hypogonadism

76. **Which of the following does not produce fasting hypoglycaemia**
    A. Galactosaemia
    B. Insulinoma
    C. Glucose-6-phosphatase deficiency
    D. Systemic carnitine deficiency

77. **Schmidt syndrome (polyglandular deficiency syndrome) is not associated with**
    A. Adrenal insufficiency
    B. Hypoparathyroidism
    C. Diabetes mellitus
    D. Phaeochromocytoma

78. **All of the following produce hirsutism with virilisation** *except*
    A. Cushing's syndrome
    B. Arrhenoblastoma
    C. Malignant adrenal hyperplasia
    D. Congenital adrenal hyperplasia

79. **Erythropoietin is secreted from**
    A. Mesenchymal tumours
    B. Cerebellar haemangioblastoma
    C. Juxtaglomerular tumour
    D. Lymphoma

80. **Turner's syndrome is not associated with**
    A. Shield-like chest
    B. Aortic incompetence
    C. Bilateral cubitus valgus
    D. Webbing of neck

81. **Melatonin is clinically used in**
    A. Pituitary tumour
    B. Decompression sickness
    C. High-altitude pulmonary oedema
    D. Jet lag

82. **POEMS syndrome aggregates polyneuropathy, organomegaly, M-proteins, skin changes and**
    A. Enlarged pituitary gland
    B. Empyema thoracis
    C. Endocrinopathy
    D. Endocarditis

83. **Sildenafil (Viagra) should be used with caution in**
    A. Retinitis pigmentosa
    B. Diabetes mellitus
    C. Endogenous depression
    D. Hypertension

Ans: 75-C 76-A 77-D 78-A 79-B 80-B 81-D 82-C 83-A

84. **Vanillylmandelic acid (VMA) excretion is increased in urine in**
   - A. Conn's syndrome
   - B. Congenital adrenal hyperplasia
   - C. Testicular feminisation syndrome
   - D. Phaeochromocytoma

85. **Commonest cause of thyrotoxicosis is**
   - A. Multinodular goitre
   - B. Hashimoto's thyroiditis
   - C. Graves' disease
   - D. Well-differentiated carcinoma

86. **In pregnancy, antithyroid treatment of choice is**
   - A. Radio-active iodine
   - B. Carbimazole
   - C. Subtotal thyroidectomy
   - D. Corticosteroid

87. **Charcot joint in diabetes mellitus commonly affects**
   - A. Hip
   - B. Shoulder
   - C. Knee
   - D. Foot

88. **Osmoreceptors are present in**
   - A. Atria
   - B. Kidney
   - C. Anterior hypothalamus
   - D. Adrenal cortex

89. **The prostaglandins were first demonstrated in**
   - A. CSF
   - B. Urine
   - C. Semen
   - D. Blood

90. **Which is considered to be an endocrine organ**
   - A. Skin
   - B. Ciliary body
   - C. Small intestine
   - D. Breast

91. **Epiphyseal dysgenesis is seen in**
   - A. Hypoparathyroidism
   - B. Secondary hyperparathyroidism
   - C. Cushing's syndrome
   - D. Hypothyroidism

92. **Commonest site of insulinoma is in the pancreatic**
   - A. Tail
   - B. Head
   - C. Body
   - D. Same incidence everywhere

93. **In Somogyi phenomenon commonly associated with type 2 diabetes mellitus, the dose of insulin should be**
   - A. Increased
   - B. Stopped
   - C. Decreased
   - D. Needs no change

Ans: 84-D 85-C 86-B 87-D 88-C 89-C 90-C 91-D 92-D 93-C

94. Miglitol used in diabetes mellitus falls under category of drugs like
    - A. Alpha-glucosidase inhibitor
    - B. Thiazolidinediones
    - C. Sulphonylureas
    - D. Biguanides

95. Thyromegaly may develop from all *except*
    - A. Chlorpromazine
    - B. Lithium
    - C. Phenylbutazone
    - D. PAS

96. In the Klinefelter's syndrome
    - A. All the patients are infertile
    - B. Plasma FSH is elevated
    - C. There may be shield-like chest
    - D. Testes and breast atrophy

97. Which of the following is not a recognised feature of myxoedema
    - A. Ascites
    - B. Cerebellar ataxia
    - C. Increased incidence of pernicious anaemia
    - D. Thyroid acropachy

98. Percussion myoedema is characteristic of
    - A. Acromegaly
    - B. Hypoparathyroidism
    - C. Sheehan's syndrome
    - D. Hypothyroidism

99. Anorexia nervosa is not associated with
    - A. Hypokalaemia
    - B. Primary amenorrhoea
    - C. Exclusively in females
    - D. Low FSH and LH

100. 'Blubbery' lips are characteristic of
    - A. Mucosal neuroma syndrome (MEN type III)
    - B. McCune-Albright syndrome
    - C. Osteogenesis imperfecta
    - D. Schmidt syndrome (polyglandular deficiency syndrome)

101. Priapism may be a side effect of
    - A. Reserpine
    - B. Octreotide
    - C. Methaqualone
    - D. Trazodone

102. Which of the following is false regarding prerequisites of oral glucose tolerance test
    - A. Restricted carbohydrate diet, 72 hours before test
    - B. Patient will take 75 g of glucose orally during the test
    - C. Fasting overnight
    - D. Should not smoke during the test

Ans: 94-A 95-A 96-B 97-D 98-D 99-C 100-A 101-D 102-A

103. **Orlistat is used to treat**
    A. Diabetic neuropathy
    B. Obesity
    C. Pseudohypoparathyroidism
    D. Anorexia nervosa

104. **Prolonged ingestion of iodine can produce goitre, and is known as**
    A. Jod-Basedow effect
    B. Sick euthyroid syndrome
    C. Wolf-Chaikoff effect
    D. Thyrotoxicosis factitia

105. **Priapism may be encountered in all *except***
    A. Spinal cord injury
    B. Alprostadil therapy
    C. Sickle cell anaemia
    D. Autonomic neuropathy

106. **Seminal emission may be absent in all *except***
    A. Phentolamine therapy
    B. Parasympathetic denervation
    C. Retrograde ejaculation
    D. Androgen deficiency

107. **Advanced maternal age is a predisposing factor in**
    A. Turner's syndrome
    B. Ataxia-telangiectasia
    C. Klinefelter's syndrome
    D. True hermaphroditism

108. **Karyotype 47, XYY is**
    A. True hermaphroditism
    B. Supermale
    C. Klinefelter's syndrome
    D. Gonadal dysgenesis

109. **Commonest cause of 'ambiguous genitalia' in newborn is**
    A. Congenital adrenal hyperplasia
    B. True hermaphroditism
    C. Testicular ferminisation syndrome
    D. Pseudohermaphroditism

110. **Hurthle cells are pathognomonic of**
    A. Pemphigus
    B. Pinealoma
    C. Hashimoto's thyroiditis
    D. Insulinoma

111. **Psammoma bodies are seen in all *except***
    A. Papillary carcinoma of thyroid
    B. Meningioma
    C. Papillary serous cystadenoma of ovary
    D. Carcinoma of body of pancreas

Ans: 103-B 104-C 105-D 106-B 107-C 108-B 109-A 110-C 111-D

112. **In a male subject, if ovulation causes testicular pain, the diagnosis is**
    A. Gonadal dysgenesis
    B. True hermaphroditism
    C. Testicular feminisation syndrome
    D. Pseudohermaphroditism

113. **A female with negative Barr body and having lymphoedema of hand and foot is diagnostic of**
    A. 21-hydroxylase deficiency   B. Karotype 47, XXY
    C. Noonan syndrome   D. Karyotype 45, XO

114. **Persistent muscular weakness is characteristic of**
    A. Conn's syndrome   B. Acromegaly
    C. Hyperparathyroidism   D. Myxoedema

115. **Galactorrhoea may be produced by all** *except*
    A. Reserpine   B. Butyrophenones
    C. Verapamil   D. Gemfibrozil

116. **Which of the following augments growth hormone release**
    A. Glucocorticoids   B. Somatostatin
    C. Stress   D. Obesity

117. **Syndrome of inappropriate antidiuretic hormone (SIADH) may be seen in all** *except*
    A. Guillain-Barré syndrome
    B. Subacute bacterial endocarditis
    C. Myxoedema
    D. Bronchogenic carcinoma

14

Geriatric Medicine

1. Causes of 'falls' in old age include all *except*
   - A. Depression
   - B. Cognitive impairment
   - C. Taking digoxin
   - D. Postural hypotension

2. Which of the following drugs may be responsible for 'falls' in the elderly
   - A. Cetrizine
   - B. Leflunomide
   - C. Acarbose
   - D. Prazosin

3. Urinary incontinence in the elderly may be due to all *except*
   - A. Irritable bowel syndrome
   - B. Stool impaction
   - C. Atrophic vaginitis
   - D. Dementia

4. All of the following drugs may cause transient incontinence of urine *except*
   - A. Desimipramine
   - B. Spironolactone
   - C. Pseudoephedrine
   - D. Benztropine

5. Which is false regarding cardiovascular changes in old age
   - A. Reduced pulse pressure
   - B. Widened aortic arch on X-ray
   - C. Increased risk of atrial fibrillations
   - D. Systolic hypertension

6. Which is not true regarding change in immune system in the elderly
   - A. False negative PPD response
   - B. ↓ T cell function
   - C. ↓ Autoantibodies
   - D. ↓ Bone marrow reserve

7. All are endocrinal changes in old age *except*
   - A. ↓ Renin
   - B. ↓ Vitamin D absorption
   - C. ↓ ADH
   - D. ↓ Thyroxine clearance

8. Which is not a physiological effect of aging
   - A. ↑ Residual volume of lung
   - B. ↑ Compliance of lung
   - C. ↓ Stroke volume
   - D. ↓ Insulin sensitivity

Ans: 1-C 2-D 3-A 4-B 5-A 6-C 7-C 8-B

9. The treatment of choice of urinary incontinence in the elderly is
   A. Prostatectomy
   B. Toilet training
   C. Oxybutynin
   D. Surgery to reduce detrusor overactivity

10. Effects of aging on drug metabolism are due to all *except*
    A. ↓ Lean body mass
    B. ↓ Renal excretion
    C. ↓ Plasma binding
    D. ↑ Hepatic first-pass metabolism

11. All of the following laboratory data are essentially unchanged in old age in comparison to reference ranges *except*
    A. Serum LDH
    B. Serum K$^+$
    C. Serum Na$^+$
    D. Serum amylase

12. In the aged, all of the following are raised in comparison to reference ranges *except*
    A. Serum alkaline phosphatase
    B. Serum globulin
    C. Serum uric acid
    D. Total leucocyte count

13. The presence of which of the following in an elderly does not imply significance
    A. Fourth heart sound
    B. Ejection click
    C. Systolic murmurs of pulmonary stenosis
    D. Third heart sound

14. Which of the following should arouse suspicion of underlying disease in a person over 70 years
    A. Loss of vibration sensation
    B. Presence of palmomental reflex
    C. Loss of ankle jerk
    D. Astereognosis

15. Alzheimer's disease is treated with
    A. Trihydroaminoacridine
    B. Amantadine
    C. Lubeluzole
    D. Donazepril

16. All of the following are age-related changes in physiologic function *except*
    A. Decreased susceptibility to hypothermia
    B. Increased T-suppressor cells
    C. Increased autoimmunity
    D Decline in baroreceptor reflex

Ans: 9-B 10-D 11-B 12-D 13-A 14-D 15-D 16-A

15

Radiology

1. In a chest X-ray PA view, the tube-film distance should be
   - A. 3 feet
   - B. 4 feet
   - C. 6 feet
   - D. 8 feet

2. 'Air bronchogram' in chest X-ray is classically seen in
   - A. Pleural effusion
   - B. Consolidation
   - C. Bronchogenic carcinoma
   - D. Emphysema

3. In pleural effusion, minimal amount of collection for X-ray detection is
   - A. 50 ml
   - B. 80 ml
   - C. 150 ml
   - D. 300 ml

4. All of the following produce unilateral hypertranslucency in X-ray *except*
   - A. Atrophy of pectoral muscle
   - B. Lung cyst
   - C. Bullae
   - D. Collapse of the lung

5. Honeycombing in chest X-ray is seen in all *except*
   - A. Bronchial adenoma
   - B. Tuberous sclerosis
   - C. Extrinsic allergic alveolitis
   - D. Bronchiectasis

6. Shifting of trachea to same side is seen in X-ray plate of
   - A. Mesothelioma of pleura
   - B. Agenesis of lung
   - C. Consolidation
   - D. Empyema thoracis

7. Miliary mottlings may be seen in
   - A. Klebsiella pneumonia
   - B. Staphylococcal pneumonia
   - C. Legionnaires' pneumonia
   - D. Chickenpox pneumonia

8. J-shaped sella turcica is seen in
   - A. Hurler's disease
   - B. Histiocytosis-X disease
   - C. Pinealoma
   - D. Prolactinoma

Ans: 1-C 2-B 3-D 4-D 5-A 6-B 7-D 8-A

9. **Geographic skull is characteristic of**
   A. Cretinism
   B. Fragile-X syndrome
   C. Multiple myeloma
   D. Hand-Schuller-Christian disease

10. **Hilar dance in fluoroscopy is diagnostic of**
   A. Patent ductus arteriosus
   B. Aortic incompetence
   C. Atrial septal defect
   D. Coarctation of aorta

11. **'String sign of Kantor' in barium meal X-ray of GI tract suggests**
   A. Carcinoid syndrome
   B. Diverticulosis
   C. Crohn's disease
   D. Irritable bowel syndrome

12. **Double bubble sign is diagnostic of**
   A. Duodenal atresia
   B. Congenital hypertrophic pyloric stenosis
   C. Jejunal atresia
   D. Pancreas divisum

13. **In barium enema, thumbprinting of colon is characteristically seen in**
   A. Ulcerative colitis
   B. Ischaemic colitis
   C. Pseudomembranous colitis
   D. Angiodysplasia of colon

14. **Ring shadow in IVP clinches the diagnosis of**
   A. Papillary necrosis
   B. Cortical necrosis
   C. Hypernephroma
   D. Tubular necrosis

15. **CT scan of brain may reveal ring shadows in all *except***
   A. Tuberculoma
   B. Brain abscess
   C. Meningioma
   D. Neurocysticercosis

16. **Calcification of diaphragmatic pleura is characteristic of**
   A. Silicosis
   B. Tuberculosis
   C. Histoplasmosis
   D. Asbestosis

17. **Water lily sign in chest X-ray is pathognomonic of**
   A. Encysted pleural effusion
   B. Congenital cystic disease of lung
   C. Hydatid cyst
   D. Cystic fibrosis

18. **Calcification of meniscal cartilage is common in**
   A. Rheumatoid arthritis
   B. Hypoparathyroidism
   C. Pseudogout
   D. Renal osteodystrophy

Ans: 9-D 10-C 11-C 12-A 13-B 14-A 15-C 16-D 17-C 18-C

19. **Trummerfeld zone in X-ray of long bones is classically seen in**

   A. Scurvy
   B. Acromegaly
   C. Rickets
   D. Down's syndrome

20. **Rib notching at lower border in chest X-ray is characteristic of**

   A. Hyperparathyroidism
   B. Neurofibromatosis
   C. Coarctation of aorta
   D. Multiple myeloma

21. **Calcification of interspinous ligament is diagnostic of**

   A. Reiter's syndrome
   B. Still's disease
   C. Hyperparathyroidism
   D. Ankylosing spondylitis

22. **Oligaemic lung field in chest X-ray is caused by all *except***

   A. Truncus arteriosus
   B. Patent ductus arteriosus
   C. Fallot's tetralogy
   D. Pericardial effusion

23. **Calcification of intervertebral disc in pathognomonic of**

   A. Renal osteodystrophy
   B. Osteopetrosis
   C. Carcinoid syndrome
   D. Alcaptonuria

24. **All are contraindications of MRI scan, if the patient has the following *except***

   A. Cochlear implant
   B. Prosthetic heart valve
   C. Ventriculoarterial shunt for hydrocephalus
   D. Pacemaker

25. **MRI scan of brain is preferred over CT scan in all *except***

   A. Calcification within a lesion
   B. Leukodystrophies
   C. Posterior fossa tumours
   D. Multiple sclerosis

26. **Positive 'sniff test' on fluoroscopy clinches the diagnosis of**

   A. Sympathetic palsy
   B. Trigeminal nerve palsy
   C. Phrenic nerve palsy
   D. Olfactory nerve palsy

27. **Irregular filling defect of oesophagus in barium swallow is seen in all *except***

   A. Oesophageal varices
   B. Gastro-oesophageal reflux disease
   C. Monilial oesophagitis
   D. Diffuse oesophageal spasm

Ans: 19-A 20-C 21-D 22-B 23-D 24-C 25-A 26-C 27-B

28. Osteosclerosis is characteristic feature of all *except*
    A. Marble bone disease
    B. Fluorosis
    C. Secondary deposits from prostatic carcinoma
    D. Non-Hodgkin's lymphoma

29. Which of the following does not fit in the barium enema findings of irritable bowel syndrome
    A. Accentuated haustrations
    B. Multiple, small ulcers
    C. Tubular appearance of the descending colon
    D. Spasticity of sigmoid colon

30. Which is false regarding Chilaiditi's syndrome
    A. Needs immediate operation in majority
    B. Mimics pneumoperitoneum
    C. Detected accidentally on straight X-ray of abdomen
    D. Bowel is interposed between liver and diaphragm

31. In X-ray, which of the following is not characteristic of rheumatoid arthritis
    A. Juxta-articular osteopenia   B. Loss of articular cartilage
    C. Pencil-in-cup deformity   D. Bone erosions

32. Basal ganglia calcification in CT scan is not a feature of
    A. Toxoplasmosis   B. Hyperparathyroidism
    C. Pseudohypoparathyroidism   D. Carbon monoxide poisoning

33. Thorotrast used in radiology is a carcinogen of
    A. Urinary bladder   B. Stomach
    C. Liver   D. Ovary

34. Flask-shaped lower end of femur is characteristic of
    A. Gaucher's disease   B. Sarcoidosis
    C. Osteopetrosis   D. Hunter's syndrome

35. All may have osteoblastic lesion *except*
    A. Carcinoid metastasis   B. Breast malignancy
    C. Prostatic malignancy   D. Malignancy of stomach

36. 'Face of the giant Panda' sign in MRI brain is often diagnostic of
    A. Hydrocephalus   B. Alzheimer's disease
    C. Huntington chorea   D. Wilson's disease

Ans: 28-D 29-B 30-A 31-C 32-B 33-C 34-A 35-D 36-D

Genetics and Immunity

1. **Programmed cell death is popularly known as**
   - A. Apoptosis
   - B. Atopy
   - C. Necrosis
   - D. Gangrene

2. **Amniocentesis is usually performed at**
   - A. 8 weeks
   - B. 12 weeks
   - C. 16 weeks
   - D. 24 weeks

3. **TNF-α is produced by all *except***
   - A. T cells
   - B. Monocyte
   - C. B cells
   - D. Macrophages

4. **All of the following are B cell disorder immunodeficiency states *except***
   - A. Wiskott-Aldrich syndrome
   - B. Di George's syndrome
   - C. X-linked agammaglobulinaemia
   - D. Selective IgA deficiency

5. **HLA association of SLE is**
   - A. DR2
   - B. DR4
   - C. DR1
   - C. DR3

6. **Pyrimidines include all of the following *except***
   - A. Cytosine
   - B. Guanine
   - C. Thymine
   - D. Uracil

7. **All are single gene disorders *except***
   - A. Polyposis coli
   - B. Sickle-cell anaemia
   - C. Turner's syndrome
   - D. Alport's syndrome

8. **X-linked disorders include all *except***
   - A. Cystic fibrosis
   - B. Duchenne's muscular dystrophy
   - C. Haemophilia
   - D. Nephrogenic diabetes mellitus

Ans: 1-A 2-C 3-C 4-B 5-D 6-B 7-C 8-A

9. **Autosomal recessive disorders do not include**
   A. Ataxia-telangiectasia
   B. Tuberous sclerosis
   C. Homocystinuria
   D. Gaucher's disease

10. **Trisomy 13 is**
    A. Crouzon's syndrome
    B. Patau's syndrome
    C. Marfan's syndrome
    D. Edward's syndrome

11. **Diseases associated with triplet repeat sequences include all** *except*
    A. Friedreich's ataxia
    B. Fragile-X syndrome
    C. Huntington's disease
    D. Refsum's disease

12. **All of the following are genetic disorders associated with chromosome 19 abnormality** *except*
    A. Myotonic dystrophy
    B. Familial hypercholesterolaemia
    C. Prader-Willi syndrome
    D. Leprechaunism

13. **Transferrin has half-life of**
    A. 1–2 days
    B. 3–4 days
    C. 5–7 days
    D. 8–9 days

14. **Which is not included in mitochondrial DNA abnormality**
    A. Kearns-Sayre syndrome
    B. Leber's optic atrophy
    C. Myoclonic epilepsy
    D. Parkinson's disease

15. **Disorder in haemochromatosis lies in chromosome number**
    A. 3
    B. 6
    C. 16
    D. 22

16. **Which is not an X-linked dominant disorder**
    A. G6PD deficiency
    B. Orofaciodigital syndrome
    C. Vitamin D resistant rickets
    D. Fabry's disease

17. **Point mutations are the cause for development of all** *except*
    A. Sickle-cell anaemia
    B. Cystic fibrosis
    C. Diabetes mellitus
    D. β-thalassaemia

18. **Fragile-X syndrome has all the following features** *except*
    A. Large testes
    B. Prognathism
    C. Ventricular septal defect
    D. Mental retardation

Ans: 9-B 10-B 11-D 12-C 13-D 14-C 15-B 16-A 17-C 18-C

19. **Arrest of mitosis by colchicine occurs in**
    A. Prophase
    B. Metaphase
    C. Anaphase
    D. Telophase

20. **Which determining factor is produced by SRY-gene**
    A. Testes
    B. Gut
    C. Ovary
    D. Brain

21. **'Lyonisation' indicates inactivation of chromosome**
    A. X
    B. Autosomes
    C. X and Y both
    D. Y

22. **Which of the following is not an autoimmune disorder**
    A. Pemphigus vulgaris
    B. Antiphospholipid syndrome
    C. Wilson's disease
    D. Hashimoto's thyroiditis

23. **Which of the following immunoglobulins has longest half-life**
    A. IgA
    B. IgE
    C. IgM
    D. IgG

24. **Which of the following is not a monogenic disorder**
    A. Achondroplasia
    B. Schizophrenia
    C. Myotonia dystrophica
    D. Malignant hyperthermia

Ans: 19-B 20-A 21-A 22-C 23-D 24-B